The ORGASM ANSWER GUIDE

The ORGASM
ANSWER GUIDE

Barry R. Komisaruk

Beverly Whipple

Sara Nasserzadeh

Carlos Beyer-Flores

The Johns Hopkins University Press | Baltimore

© 2010 The Johns Hopkins University Press
All rights reserved. Published 2010
Printed in the United States of America on acid-free paper
2   4   6   8   9   7   5   3   1

The Johns Hopkins University Press
2715 North Charles Street
Baltimore, Maryland 21218-4363
www.press.jhu.edu

Library of Congress Cataloging-in-Publication Data

The orgasm answer guide / Barry R. Komisaruk ... [et al.].
p. cm.
Includes bibliographical references.
ISBN-13: 978-0-8018-9395-7 (hardcover : alk. paper)
ISBN-10: 0-8018-9395-X (hardcover : alk. paper)
ISBN-13: 978-0-8018-9396-4 (pbk. : alk. paper)
ISBN-10: 0-8018-9396-8 (pbk. : alk. paper)
1. Orgasm—Popular works. I. Komisaruk, Barry R.
QP251.O74 2009
613.9'6—dc22   2009009804

A catalog record for this book is available from the British Library.

Special discounts are available for bulk purchases of this book. For more information, please contact Special Sales
at 410-516-6936 or specialsales@press.jhu.edu.

The Johns Hopkins University Press uses environmentally friendly book materials, including recycled text paper that is composed of at least 30 percent post-consumer waste, whenever possible. All of our book papers are acid-free, and our jackets and covers are printed on
paper with recycled content.

Contents

Two   Women's Orgasms

Three   Men's Orgasms

Four Hows and Whys of Orgasm

Five Orgasms and Health

Six   The Geography of the Female Orgasm

Seven Orgasms and Relationships

Preface

WHEN YOU WORK IN the field of sexual health, you are asked a lot of questions. Sometimes you know the answer, sometimes you need to call on colleagues for advice. This book is a combination of our knowledge and the assistance we have received from many people. We are grateful to all those who have posed questions to us throughout the years and especially to the following people, who helped us before and during the writing of this book: Rachel Abrams, John Bancroft, Edwin Belzer, Wendy Birbano, Karen Brash-McGreer, Maria Cruz Rodriguez del Cerro, Arlene Feldman, Eleni Frangos, David Goldmeier, Gabriela Gonzalez-Mariscal, Cynthia Graham, Serin Kelami, Harvey Kliman, Roy Levin, Christine McGinn, Angelica Montiel-Breton, Michael Perelman, Martha Rivera, Jay Rosenblatt, Kenneth Ray Stubbs, Alexander Tsiaras, Mary Ann Ulrich, Nan Wise, and Kevan Wylie. Without their assistance, this book would never have been possible. We also acknowledge, with special thanks, our editor, Vincent J. Burke, for his continuous encouragement, support, thoughtfulness, and expert advice and help. We offer our sincere gratitude to Linda Strange, our copyeditor, for her excellent unruffling of our text.

We think the diversity of our professional and personal backgrounds helps make the book both readable and comprehensive. Professionally, among the four authors we have some level of expertise in virtually every aspect of sexual health related to orgasm. Personally, we are a diverse religious and cultural mix—Christian, Jewish, and Muslim; American, Middle Eastern, and Mexican.

After numerous conversations among the four of us, we settled on eighty or so questions that represent what we think you are curious about. Some of our answers are brief, others more detailed. We tried to answer the questions without getting bogged down in scientific details, but we also tried not to leave out important information--even if it meant including the occasional medical term. We tested the manuscript on both experts and non-experts and, we hope, have produced a book that satisfies both groups.

Researching and writing a book takes you away from the ones you love for far too many hours of the day. For their understanding and support, Barry thanks his sons, Adam and Kevin, and, in remembrance, his wife, Carrie. Beverly thanks her husband, Jim, children, Allen and Susan, and grandchildren, Kayla, Travis, Valerie, William, and Elyse. Sara thanks her husband, Pejman Azarmina. Carlos thanks his wife, Josefina, and daughters, Maria Emilia and Gaby.

The ORGASM ANSWER GUIDE

One

About Orgasms

What are orgasms?

As simple as this question sounds, and as obvious as the answer may seem to most of us, defining "orgasm" can prove difficult. In some ways, it is as difficult to define "orgasm" as it is to describe how something tastes.

Let's begin to explore the meaning of the word *orgasm* by looking at its linguistic origin, the Greek word *orgasmos*, which is defined as "to swell as with moisture, be excited or eager" (*Oxford English Dictionary*). Alternatively, we could use the more technical definition offered in the Kinsey Reports: "The expulsive discharge of neuromuscular tensions at the peak of sexual response." An even more technical description was offered by the research team of Masters and Johnson: "A brief episode of physical release from the vasocongestion and myotonic increment developed in response to sexual stimuli."

Perhaps the most interesting of all characterizations is the one that was offered by John Money, who, with his colleagues, wrote the following description of orgasm: "The zenith of sexuoerotic experience that men and women characterize subjectively as voluptuous rapture or ecstasy. It occurs simultaneously in the brain/mind and the pelvic genitalia. Irrespective of its locus of onset, the occurrence of orgasm is contingent upon reciprocal intercommunication between neural networks in the brain, above, and the pelvic genitalia, below, and it does not survive their disconnection by the severance of the spinal cord. However, it is able to survive even extensive trauma at either end."

So, what are orgasms? Here is our broad definition: an orgasm is a buildup of pleasurable body sensations and excitement to a peak intensity that then releases tensions and creates a feeling of satisfaction and relaxation.

Do men and women have the same sensations during an orgasm?

NOBODY CAN REALLY FEEL someone else's pleasure, so comparisons of the sort implied by this question are difficult to make. However, the following experiment was a clever way of getting at the question. Researchers Vance and Wagner, in 1976, asked college students to write descriptions of their own orgasms, and a group of judges tried to guess which descriptions were written by men and which by women. The judges were a mix of female and male obstetrician-gynecologists, psychologists, and medical students. Before submitting the descriptions to the judges, the researchers substituted gender-neutral words for gender-specific words in the students' written descriptions (such as *genitalia* for *penis* or *vagina*) to intentionally conceal the sex of the writers.

The researchers found that the judges were "unable to distinguish the sex of a person from that person's written description of his or her orgasm."

The students' descriptions are vivid, as demonstrated by the following quotations, selected at random from the responses of six of the forty-eight participants in the study:

- A sudden feeling of lightheadedness followed by an intense feeling of relief and elation. A rush. Intense muscular spasms of the whole body. Sense of euphoria followed by deep peace and relaxation.
- Feels like tension building up until you think it can't build up any more, then release. The orgasm is both the highest point of tension and the release almost at the same time. Also feeling contractions in the genitals. Tingling all over.
- There is a great release of tensions that have built up in the prior stages of sexual activity. This release is extremely pleasurable and exciting. The feeling seems to be centered in the genital region. It is extremely intense and exhilarating. There is a loss of muscular control as the pleasure mounts and you almost cannot go on. You almost don't want to go on. This is followed by the climax and refractory states.
- The period when the orgasm takes place—a loss of a real feeling for the surroundings except for the other person. The movements are spontaneous and intense.
- A heightened feeling of excitement with severe muscular tension especially through the back and legs, rigid straightening of the entire body for about five seconds, and a strong and general relaxation and very tired relieved feeling.
- Basically it's an enormous buildup of tension, anxiety, strain followed by a period of total oblivion to sensation then a tremendous expulsion of the buildup with a feeling of wonderfulness and relief.

One reason that men and women *may* experience similar feelings during orgasm is related to two of the primary body parts involved in orgasm: the penis and clitoris. These body parts are *homologous*, meaning that they both originate from the same tissue in the developing embryo. Throughout life, the spinal cord and brain are connected to the penis and clitoris by the same nerve route—the pudendal nerve (actually, a pair of pudendal nerves). So, while we don't know the answer to the question with certainty, there are reasons to suspect that orgasms may feel generally similar for men and women.

Why don't all my orgasms feel the same?

GENITALS ARE CONNECTED TO several different pairs of nerves, with each pair of nerves servicing (that is, carrying nerve impulses from) a different part of the person's genital areas. Stimulating different combinations of the nerves produces different combinations of sensations. Depending on the parts of the genitals that are stimulated and the relative intensity and pattern of the stimulation, orgasms may feel very different from one time to another.

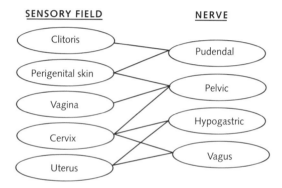

Nerves carrying information between the female genital regions and the brain. Each of the four named nerves is a pair of nerves--one on the left side, one on the right. Some genital regions use more than one pair of nerves to communicate with the brain, as shown by the connecting lines in the diagram. Three of the nerve pairs (the pudendal, pelvic, and hypogastric) travel to the spinal cord, where the sensations are then transmitted to the brain. The pair of vagus nerves, however, travel directly to the brain, bypassing the spinal cord.

For a woman, the sensory quality of an orgasm depends on where the stimulation occurs: the clitoris, vagina, or cervix. The clitoris is connected mainly to the pudendal nerves, the vagina mainly to the pelvic nerves, and the cervix mainly to the hypogastric, pelvic, and vagus nerves. Although stimulating each of these genital regions may by itself produce orgasms, the combined stimulation of two or three regions has an additive effect, producing a more encompassing orgasm, or what is described as "blended orgasm."

In a man, the pudendal nerves carry nerve impulses from the penile skin and scrotum, and the hypogastric nerves carry nerve impulses from the testicles and prostate gland. So, stimulation of these two nerve groups may cause somewhat different feelings.

For many people, their "erogenous zones" extend beyond the genitals. The location of these zones is amazingly diverse and highly individualistic. Stimulation of an individual's "personal erogenous zones" can greatly affect the intensity of his or her orgasms. In addition to sensory factors, orgasms are often affected by cognitive, psychological, and pharmacological factors—such as distraction, worry, relaxation, medications, and the like.

What are multiple orgasms?

ORGASMS THAT OCCUR IN close succession, within a few seconds to a few minutes apart, are often referred to as "multiple orgasms." Although there is no consensus among researchers about what defines multiple orgasms, we do know that some individuals experience orgasms multiple times in a relatively brief period. Multiple orgasms are more frequently discussed in relation to women's sexual responses, but men can experience them as well. Indeed, as early as 2968 BC, in China, there were writings that described men's multiple orgasms.

What is anorgasmia?

THE WORD *ANORGASMIA* MEANS "a lack of orgasm." This condition occurs in both men and women.

In men, anorgasmia is usually called "male orgasmic dysfunction," and both biological ("organic") and psychological factors may contribute to this condition. The current definition of male orgasmic dysfunction is "a spectrum of disorders ranging from delayed ejaculation to complete inability to ejaculate ('anejaculation'), and retrograde ejaculation." Any disease, drug, or surgical procedure that interferes with the normal functioning of the brain, spinal cord, or nerves can result in male orgasmic dysfunction. One of the main classes of drugs that inhibit orgasm is the SSRIs (selective serotonin reuptake inhibitors), which are commonly prescribed for depression.

Women's anorgasmia, or "orgasmic disorder," is defined as "either a lack of orgasm, markedly diminished intensity of orgasmic sensations or marked delay of orgasm from any kind of stimulation." Professionals in the field classify female anorgasmia into three types: primary, secondary, and situational anorgasmia. The diagnosis of "primary anorgasmia" applies to a woman who has never experienced an orgasm by any means of stimulation. "Secondary anorgasmia" refers to the case in which a woman was previously orgasmic but currently is anorgasmic. "Situational anorgasmia" relates to the conditions under which a woman may or may not experience orgasm—such as being able to experience orgasm by masturbation but not with a partner. According to researcher Raymond Rosen, anorgasmia is a common problem that affects an estimated 24 to 37 percent of women.

Therapy for anorgasmia includes a combination of a check-up by a medical professional (reviewing the history of medications and conducting necessary tests) and the use of "behavioral therapies." Behavioral strategies have proven very effective for both men and women. Such strategies include "sensate focus exercises" (to gradually build up one's comfort with intimate physical contact), directed masturbation (that is, masturbation under the advice of a therapist) with or without a vibrator, Kegel exercises (to strengthen the muscles of the pelvic floor), and physical therapy. Other issues that may cause anorgasmia and that may be treated by behavioral therapy include anxiety, a past history of sexual abuse or trauma, problems in communication with the sexual partner, and issues of trust of the partner.

The simplest, and perhaps most helpful, treatment for the largest number of people who experience anorgasmia may be for health care providers to ask questions and offer information. Orgasms can be elicited from a variety of body regions, including the penis, clitoris, vagina, G spot, cervix, prostate, nipples, breasts, anus—as well as through visual and auditory stimulation and mental imagery. Here's an important point: while you can be stimulated erotically by your partner, your partner can't "give" you an orgasm. You are in control of your own feelings, including your orgasms. And even if you don't experience an orgasm, you can nevertheless derive great pleasure and satisfaction from a positive sexual encounter.

At what age do orgasms begin?

ALTHOUGH MOST PEOPLE CAN experience orgasms fairly often by the age of ten to fifteen, there is some debate as to when a person is *first* able to experience an orgasm. In the past half-century, numerous psychologists and anthropologists have described a wide array of sexual responses in children, including orgasm. Indeed, children of both sexes often explore their genitals, and such tactile self-stimulation can cause muscle reactions that are difficult to distinguish from orgasm in adult subjects. However, no well-controlled studies—that is, no rigorously conducted scientific studies—on children's sexual responses, including orgasm, have been reported in recent years. The nerve (neural) network needed for many sexual responses is present and functional from the time of early childhood, and penile erection can even occur in the human fetus (that is, within the uterus). However, when young boys experience what seem to be orgasm-like responses, these responses are not accompanied by ejaculation, which requires the presence of androgens (such as testosterone), sex hormones that are not present in sufficient quantities for ejaculation before puberty.

Do orgasms end at a certain age?

MANY STUDIES ON AGING and sexual behavior have found a clear pattern of an overall decline of sexual function beginning when people enter their thirties or forties, but some people can experience orgasms past the age of ninety. As they age, both men and, more often, women experience the loss of their lifelong sexual partner due to death or illness, a loss that often leads to a decrease in sexual activity.

Some studies suggest that, for women, the ability to become sexually aroused remains as the individual ages. However, many women experience declines of desire, frequency of intercourse (coitus), and frequency of orgasm as they age (often well in advance of menopause). In a recent study of older women (average age was eighty-one years), only 18 percent were still sexually active, mainly by masturbation. There is good evidence that when older women have sexual problems, some of the causes are related to decreases in the secretion of the sex steroids—estrogen and androgen. For example, vaginal dryness and a condition known as dyspareunia (painful intercourse) are due to low levels of estrogen (which is correctable by vaginal estrogen therapy).

Sexual function and orgasm frequency also decline in men as they age. However, a typical older man (average age in the eighties) is twice as likely to be sexually active as a woman of a similar age (41 percent of men versus 18 percent of women). The most common type of sexual disorder in older men is erectile dysfunction.

A comparable pattern of sexual decline and disorder accompanying aging has been observed in nonhuman animals. For example, very old rabbits still attempt to copulate despite erectile dysfunction, and they will copulate successfully after receiving Viagra.

How long does it take to reach orgasm?

DURING SEXUAL INTERCOURSE, THE amount of time before reaching orgasm varies considerably among individuals. Factors such as age, sexual experience, and certain drugs influence the time it takes to reach orgasm. Both men and women can voluntarily delay orgasm through a variety of techniques. For example, in some practices of Hinduism—such as Tantra, which puts great emphasis on sexual intercourse for religious purposes— techniques developed over hundreds of years allow some individuals to control ejaculation and orgasm. In recent years, these techniques have been incorporated into practices in the western world, through a series of books that promote increased sexual satisfaction (see, for example, books by Kenneth Ray Stubbs).

Men typically require two to ten minutes of intercourse to reach orgasm. Men who experience "delayed orgasms" may need an hour or more of stimulation. Researcher Manfred Waldinger and his colleagues proposed that men who have early (premature) ejaculation and those who have delayed ejaculation are just extremes of the normal range of variability. They proposed that any random group of men will include some with early ejaculation (occurring within two minutes of starting sexual intercourse) and others with delayed ejaculation (requiring more than one hour of active intercourse). So, lifelong early or delayed ejaculators are considered to be part of the natural variability that occurs in any population. A common characteristic of many, but not all, rapid and delayed ejaculators is their lack of control of the ejaculatory latency. By contrast, a man who is near average for the duration of intercourse before orgasm may be more capable of controlling his ejaculation.

Several studies have found that most women require a more prolonged period of stimulation before orgasm. While some women have an orgasm within thirty seconds of starting self-stimulation, most women experience orgasm after twenty minutes.

How long do orgasms normally last?

ALTHOUGH THE TIME IT takes a person to reach orgasm is highly variable for both men and women, the duration of orgasm itself is less variable, and is shorter. In one study, women's orgasms were found to last, on average, about eighteen seconds, and men's orgasms lasted about twenty-two seconds. However, in 1966, Masters and Johnson found that the duration of orgasm in women is typically about three to fifteen seconds, while orgasms in men are shorter. Multiple factors are known to influence how long an orgasm lasts, such as age, period of sexual abstinence, type of sexual stimulation, and whether the orgasm is a result of masturbation or sexual intercourse. With aging, there is a tendency for the duration of orgasms to decrease.

How often do people experience orgasm?

THE FREQUENCY OF ORGASM and attitudes toward the frequency vary greatly among individuals and cultures. Some societies have recommended restraint in sexual activity for men, because ejaculation was considered debilitating; but other societies have considered sexual activity highly beneficial for vigor and health. Researcher Havelock Ellis, in 1910, surveyed historical and religious pronouncements on the appropriate frequencies of marital coitus (and presumably orgasm) for men, and he reported the following recommendations:

- Zoroaster, Persian religious leader: once in nine days
- Hindu authorities: three to six times per month
- Solon, Athenian statesman and poet: three times per month
- The Koran: once per week
- The Talmud: once per day to once per week, depending on occupation
- Martin Luther, German founder of Protestantism: twice per week

Typically, couples have more orgasms the younger they are. Kinsey reported that men had an average intercourse frequency of four times per week when they were fifteen to twenty years of age, three times per week at age thirty, twice per week at age forty, and less than once per week at age sixty. However, studies show that some men between the ages of sixteen and thirty experience as many as twenty-five orgasms per week.

A "refractory period" just after orgasm occurs in most men, a period when they can't have another orgasm—although some men can experience multiple orgasms. A report of one such case documented six successive orgasms (with decreasing volume of semen) in less than forty minutes. The duration of the "recharge time" seems to depend on age, sexual partner, and sexual experience. The brain mechanisms involved in the refractory period have been extensively studied in laboratory animals. In laboratory rats, ejaculation is accompanied by release of the neurotransmitter GABA (gamma amino-butyric acid) from neurons (nerve cells) in the brain, a process that inhibits the activity of neurons that control sexual motivation. The neural basis for the refractory period in humans is not known.

In 1994, a study based on interviews of 436 partnered women in the United Kingdom investigated the occurrence of female orgasm during the prior three-month period. There was a clear relationship between a woman's age and the likelihood that she experienced orgasm during a sexual encounter. Of the women thirty-five to thirty-nine years old, 63 percent reported experiencing orgasms during more than half of or all of their sexual interactions with their partner. Only 21 percent of women fifty-five to fifty-nine years old reported this frequency. Five percent of the younger women, but 35 percent of the older women, had not experienced an orgasm in the past three months. The intermediate age groups were intermediate in frequency of orgasm.

Does a person inherit the ability to have orgasms?

ONE WAY OF TESTING whether a behavioral trait, of any sort, has a genetic basis—or in other words, whether it is to some extent inherited—is to compare identical twins and fraternal twins. Identical twins have the same genetic makeup, because they come from the same fertilized egg. By contrast, fraternal twins develop from two different fertilized eggs and therefore are as different from each other as are two non-twin siblings; they just happen to be born at the same time.

Researchers use the reasoning that if a particular behavioral trait occurs much more frequently in both identical twins than in both fraternal twins, then there is probably a genetic component to the trait. Of course, that evidence alone doesn't explain how the genes affect the trait. In one study that looked at whether there is a genetic basis to women's orgasms, Kate Dunn and her colleagues reported the responses to questionnaires from almost 1,400 women in the TwinsUK study group. About half of the women were identical twins and half were fraternal twins. There was considerable variability in the frequency of their orgasms during intercourse or masturbation. However, the identical twins were much more similar in their frequency of orgasm than were the fraternal twins. The authors stated: "We found that between 34% and 45% of the variation in ability to orgasm can be explained by underlying genetic variation, with little or no role for the shared environment (e.g., family environment, religion, social class, or early education). These heritability findings are in a similar range (35-60%) to other behavioural and complex traits such as migraine, blood pressure, anxiety or depression."

This conclusion is similar to that of Khytam Dawood and her colleagues, based on a questionnaire study of more than 2,000 women identified in the Australian Twin Registry. These researchers concluded that "overall, genetic influences account for approximately 31% of the variance of frequency of orgasm during sexual intercourse . . . and 51% . . . during masturbation."

Are there really "nongenital" orgasms?

ORGASMS CHARACTERISTICALLY RESULT FROM genital stimulation, but there are many accounts suggesting that nongenital stimuli can also generate feelings that have been described, by both men and women, as orgasms. Here is a partial list:

- "Thinking off" orgasms produced by mental imagery in the absence of physical stimulation. Studies of women who were "thinking off," conducted in the 1960s, were corroborated in the 1990s by some laboratory studies in which women were shown to have elevations in heart rate, blood pressure, pupil diameter, and pain thresholds that are typical of orgasm.

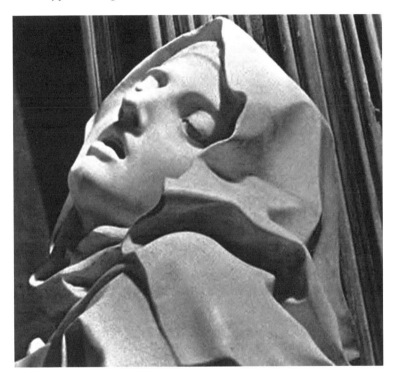

St. Teresa of Avila. Shown here is a detail of *Ecstasy of St. Teresa*, by the seventeenth-century sculptor Giovanni Lorenzo Bernini. St. Teresa of Avila is said to have been able to enter trances in which she described an ecstatic state of rapture and sweet pain in feeling union with God. The description and the facial expression shown here are similar to those characterizing orgasm, suggesting to some (but refuted by others) that she may have experienced nongenital orgasms. (Photograph courtesy Terry Ginesi)

- Orgasms experienced during meditation, as popularized by Kenneth Ray Stubbs, who provides detailed accounts of orgasmic experiences during many different types of meditation
- Orgasms experienced during prayer and meditation, as documented by William Stayton
- Orgasms produced in women and men with spinal cord injury, by their loved one caressing hypersensitive nongenital skin zones near the site of injury
- Epileptic seizures producing orgasmic auras
- "Phantom" orgasms, occurring in men and women with spinal cord injury, who feel genital orgasms in their sleep even though their injury blocks their conscious genital sensations
- "Phantom limb" orgasms, such as orgasms "felt" in an amputated foot
- Orgasms produced by stimulation of mouth, lip, breast, nipple, anus, shoulder, or toe
- Orgasms produced as a result of stimulation of *any* part of the body by the "right" person in the "right" way
- Orgasms during childbirth
- Orgasms during defecation and "forceful urination"
- Orgasms during tooth brushing by a woman with epilepsy
- Orgasms produced by direct electrical or chemical stimulation of the brain, as reported during a brief period in the 1950s before restrictions were imposed on such research
- Orgasms produced unexpectedly by electrical stimulation of the spine, initially done for pain control
- Orgasms produced by stimulation after male-to-female or female-to-male transsexual surgery
- Nongenital orgasms experienced under the influence of psychedelic drugs

Why do people sometimes look as if they are in pain at or near orgasm?

THE PARTS OF THE brain and spinal cord that control pain and orgasm overlap. This close association has some interesting consequences. For example, on the positive side, during orgasm produced by vaginal self-stimulation, women become half as sensitive to pain as they normally are (when at rest). In some cases, when surgeons were called upon to stop pain that could not be controlled by medication, they cut specific neural pathways in the spinal cord to stop the pain; as a result, however, the patients' orgasms also became blocked. Sometimes the surgery was only effective temporarily, and the pain returned six months later—but, then, so did the ability to experience orgasms!

Examination of brain activity during orgasms or during experimentally induced pain shows that at least two brain regions—the insular cortex and the anterior cingulate cortex—are active during both

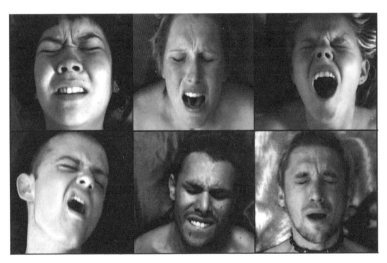

Pleasure or pain? Pain and orgasm share a curious similarity of facial expression. Two of the brain regions that are activated by pain are also activated during orgasm, perhaps accounting for the similarity of expression. (Photographs courtesy Richard Lawrence)

experiences. This raises an intriguing but as yet unanswered question: How exactly does the brain distinguish between pain and pleasure, and what is the difference between the neurons that create the sensation of pain and those that create the sensation of orgasm?

Could the two brain regions have some property that is common to both pain and pleasure, perhaps the same intense emotional *expression* (controlling the contorted facial expressions that occur during both painful anguish and impending orgasm), but separate from the different *feelings* of pain versus pleasure? It seems possible. Perhaps the pain and pleasure pathways carrying sensation through the spinal cord and brain stream along together, producing similar effects on arousal and facial expression before diverging somewhere in the brain to pass the message either to a pain-sensing part of the cortex or to a different, pleasure-sensing part of the cortex. Until this divergence occurs, perhaps the sensory activity from either the genital or the noxious stimulation passes to the brain region that generates facial expression—so that the expression is curiously similar under both conditions.

Two

Women's Orgasms

What's the difference between vaginal, cervical, and clitoral orgasms?

As the names imply, we typically refer to a "vaginal orgasm" when the primary site of stimulation is the vagina (without stimulation of the cervix) and a "cervical orgasm" when the focus of stimulation is the cervix. A "clitoral orgasm" is one in which the stimulation is specifically applied to the clitoris. Some women prefer stimulation that is confined to the vagina or cervix or both, and others prefer stimulation that is focused on the clitoris. However, some women seem to experience the greatest intensity of orgasm when the clitoris and the vagina or cervix—or all three areas—are stimulated simultaneously. Combined stimulation of all three areas activates three or four pairs of different nerves and provides a cumulative effect.

Does breast or nipple stimulation affect a woman's orgasm?

For some women, stimulation of the nipples and breasts can increase the likelihood of having an orgasm and increase its intensity. However, some women find this stimulation has either no effect or a negative effect. The orgasm-inducing effect of breast or nipple stimulation may be due to sensory activity from the breast traveling ("projecting") to some of the same neurons, in the region of the brain known as the hypothalamus, that receive sensory activity from the genitals. Because of this convergence of nerve impulses from genital and breast stimulation onto the same neurons in the hypothalamus, breast stimulation may enhance the effect of genital stimulation on orgasm.

Do Kegel exercises intensify female orgasms?

At present, there isn't enough information to answer this question. These exercises were developed for women in the 1940s by gynecologist Arnold Kegel, and this workout became popularly known as "Kegels." Kegel taught women who suffered with "urinary stress incontinence" (USI)—the leakage of urine when a woman coughs, jumps, or sneezes—how to strengthen their pelvic floor muscles. Kegel argued that his technique could avert the need for surgery, and indeed it did for most of his patients. Coincidentally, many of his patients experienced orgasm for the first time. In the decades that followed, several researchers reported that men can experience multiple orgasms when they practice contracting their pelvic floor muscles.

Kegel exercises mainly strengthen the PC (pubococcygeus) muscles, which are really a group of several muscles. In men and women, the PC muscles connect the pubic bone to the coccyx (the tailbone at the end of the spine). In other animals, this muscle group wags the tail. In humans, it supports the internal sexual organs, urethra, bladder, and rectum, preventing them from sagging. To use an analogy, the PC muscles (a flat,

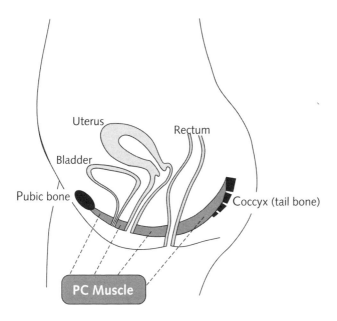

The PC (pubococcygeus) muscles. This sheet of muscles stretches between, and is attached to, the pubic bone and the coccyx. The urethra, vagina, and rectum penetrate through the muscle sheet. Kegel exercises are designed to strengthen it and prevent it from sagging.

broad sheet of muscles) are like the flexible jumping surface of a trampoline. The pubic bone at the front of the body and the coccyx at the tip of the spine are like the rigid frame of the trampoline. Kegel exercises tighten the PC muscles, ensuring that the vagina, urethra, bladder, and rectum are well supported and don't sag.

Kegel invented a device to help him evaluate the PC muscles of his female patients and to assist in training them. This instrument, called a Kegel perineometer, may have been the world's first biofeedback device.

Using the perineometer, researchers in the 1970s measured the strength of women's PC muscles in relation to their orgasmic experience. They analyzed data from 281 women who had visited their sex therapy clinic, then divided the women into three groups: those who could not experience orgasm, those who could experience orgasm from clitoral stimulation only, and those who could experience orgasm from clitoral or vaginal stimulation. The group of women who experienced orgasm with clitoral or vaginal stimulation had the strongest PC muscles, and those who could not experience orgasm had the weakest PC muscles. The group who could experience orgasm only from clitoral stimulation had intermediate muscle strength. In other words, there was a correlation between the strength of the women's pelvic muscles and their orgasmic responses. A study in 1981 reported that women who experienced female ejaculation had stronger PC muscles than women who never experienced ejaculation.

Taken together, these studies suggest that Kegel exercises probably do increase the likelihood of orgasm.

To locate your PC muscles, start to urinate with your legs apart and then stop the flow of urine. The muscles you squeeze are the PC muscles. Practice stopping the flow a few times to become familiar with the muscles. If you are interested in performing Kegel exercises, we recommend the instructions at www.mayoclinic.com/health/kegel-exercises/WO00119.

What fluids are produced before and during a woman's orgasm?

Two MAIN TYPES OF fluid are associated with women's orgasms: vaginal lubricant and female ejaculate. The clear vaginal lubricant is not secreted by glands. Instead, it seeps into the vaginal canal from blood capillaries in the vaginal lining (a process termed "transudation"), beginning as small beads and ultimately coalescing until the fluid moistens the entire inner surface of the vagina. (Incidentally, antihistamines may interfere with vaginal lubrication, as a side effect of their desired treatment for a runny nose.)

During orgasm, women may expel fluid from their urethra (the tubular structure through which urine passes out of the body), a process referred to as "female ejaculation." Female ejaculation has a controversial past. Many women reported that they underwent surgery to correct this "problem," and others reported that they inhibited their orgasms to prevent "wetting the bed." Some people are under the impression that the secreted fluid is urine. It is not. The fluid resembles dilute fat-free milk and has a sweet taste. Although the volume may seem large during an orgasm, the total amount of liquid expelled rarely exceeds one teaspoonful (five milliliters).

Several researchers chemically analyzed the fluid produced by female ejaculation and found that it contains high levels of glucose and an enzyme called prostatic acid phosphatase, and low levels of urea and creatinine. This chemical composition differs substantially from that of a woman's typical urine, which contains high levels of urea and creatinine and no prostatic acid phosphatase or glucose. A woman may experience ejaculation regularly, on rare occasions, or never. We are aware of no credible evidence that women can learn to control this process (that is, either enhance or decrease it). The important point is that female ejaculation is a normal, though not universal, process. One study suggested that perhaps all women ejaculate during orgasm, but the volume of the ejaculate is often so small that it's undetected, remaining in the urethra or passing back into the urinary bladder.

Aristotle was probably the first to write about female ejaculation, and the Greco-Roman physician and philosopher Galen is said to have known about it in the second century AD. Many others have written about female ejaculation, including the gynecologist Ernst Gräfenberg in 1950.

We should note, however, that during sexual activities and orgasm, some women may ejaculate and other women may expel urine. A review of the scientific literature that was published in 1991 found that in some women, G spot stimulation, orgasm, and female ejaculation are related (but this is certainly not universal). Other studies reported that some women experience ejaculation with orgasm in response to clitoral stimulation and some women experience ejaculation without orgasm. Most women who do experience ejaculation say that it feels pleasurable.

Why is the clitoris so sensitive after an orgasm?

ALTHOUGH INCREASED SENSITIVITY OF the clitoris is common after orgasm, there seems to be no research that specifically reveals the cause of this increased sensitivity. However, we can make an educated guess, based on what we do know about sensations during sex, at a plausible explanation.

One of the changes that a woman's body goes through when sexually aroused is the dilation (opening wider) of blood vessels. This increases the flow of blood to the genital area, resulting in swelling ("engorgement") of the clitoris. This may itself make the clitoris more sensitive to stimulation. And, in addition to the physical changes in the clitoris, the mental and emotional changes occurring in the brain increase the woman's attention to her clitoral sensations. When overdone, physical stimulation of the clitoris may become painful or even result in the clitoris becoming numb. Heightened sensitivity of the clitoris may persist after orgasm and slowly subside as the engorgement decreases over a period of minutes. During the period right after orgasm, a woman may be caught between two worlds. Her sexual intensity has diffused, but her sensory awareness may remain high. So she may now pay more attention to the sensitivity of her clitoris.

Some women say that their nipples also become very sensitive to touch after orgasm. Some like to continue the stimulation of the highly sensitized clitoris or nipples after the initial orgasm, to experience multiple orgasms. Clearly, there are major differences among women in both sensitivity and preference.

A few rare cases have been reported of women having an overly sensitive clitoris, so that even the mild friction of their clothing creates discomfort. In such cases, medical consultation is advisable.

Does body position during sex affect a woman's orgasm?

YES, BODY POSITIONS DURING vaginal intercourse can affect orgasms in women. To stimulate the G spot during vaginal intercourse (the G spot is an erogenous region just behind the pubic bone), the penis must make contact with the anterior wall of the vagina (the side of the vaginal wall closest to the belly). For most couples, the best positions for stimulating this area are: (1) the woman on top, so that she can direct the positioning of the penis in her vagina; (2) the rear entry position, in which the head of the penis can most directly contact the area of the G spot; and (3) the man on top, kneeling, so his penis will contact the anterior wall of the vagina.

To stimulate the cervix during vaginal intercourse, the couple should use a position in which there is deep penetration of the penis. One position is with the woman lying on her back with her legs elevated and around the man's back or neck. Deep penetration is more likely if the woman pulls her legs toward her body. Placing a pillow under the woman's lower back can also allow deep stimulation.

In the "coital alignment technique" (CAT), the woman lies on her back and the man lies flat on top of her, aligned as close to the woman's head as possible. In this position, the penis can stimulate the clitoris and the G spot simultaneously. Some women like to have their clitoris stimulated manually during vaginal intercourse. For these women, positions such as woman on top, either facing away from her partner (the "cowgirl" position) or facing toward her partner, can allow stimulation of the clitoris with a finger.

Certain positions are preferred by couples in which one or both partners are overweight. For an overweight man, he can sit on a chair, with the woman sitting on top of him. For the "missionary position" (man on top), it's important for the man to avoid placing all his weight on the partner. He can put his weight on his knees and hands to control the weight he puts on his partner. If the woman is overweight, she can expose her vulva and vagina by lying on her back, bending her knees and pulling them toward her belly, making penetration easier.

There are also positions that are recommended for couples in which one or both partners have a chronic illness or disability. Whipple and Welner discuss positions for vaginal intercourse and provide line drawings of suggested positions in their chapter "Sexuality Issues" in *Welner's Guide to the Care of Women with Disabilities.* Some suggested positions are the person with disability in a wheelchair, or lying on a table or bed, while the partner is standing.

Does penis size affect a woman's orgasm?

FOR MOST COUPLES, THE answer to this question is probably not. Although some women do say that the length and girth of their partner's penis is important (one study suggests that girth is far more important than length), most studies indicate that the dimensions of the penis don't affect women's overall satisfaction or probability of having an orgasm. Indeed, just as penises vary in shape and size, so too do vaginas vary in shape, size, and sensitivity among individuals. So, size preference between partners—the idea of "a good fit"—probably does not lend itself to generalizations.

Typically, if a penis is of average length (four to six inches when erect) and each partner is familiar with the pleasurable areas of the other's body, the size of the penis will probably matter less than how it is used. When a penis is larger or smaller than average, extra effort may be required with some partners to increase contact or avoid uncomfortable pressure.

Are orgasms affected by the menstrual cycle?

YES, ALTHOUGH THERE IS considerable variation among women. Some women enjoy bodily intimacy with their partner during their menstrual period, whereas others prefer not to be physically intimate during that time. Similarly, a woman's partner may be reluctant to be sexually intimate with her because of hygienic considerations, fear of causing discomfort, or cultural factors.

Researchers at Yale University reported that when a woman is not menstruating, her orgasms during sexual intercourse produce traveling wave-like uterine contractions that can suck semen into the uterus. By contrast, during menstruation, orgasms produce uterine contractions that travel in the opposite direction, which has the effect of pushing debris out of the uterus instead of sucking inward. The changing levels of hormones over the menstrual cycle play an important role in affecting the direction of these uterine contractions. This changing direction of uterine contractions could account for the observation that orgasms during menstruation may produce a surge of menstrual blood flow. The use of the Instead Softcup, which is a menstrual cup, *not* a contraceptive, may be used to collect this menstrual blood when a woman has vaginal intercourse during her period.

The research team of Morris and Udry explored differences in women's sexual activity on menstrual and nonmenstrual days, using daily report data from eighty-five women and their spouses over about a hundred days. They concluded that in their group of respondents, the desire for intercourse and the frequency of intercourse and orgasm decreased during menstruation. The women responded to increases in their husband's sexual frustration at this time by providing more noncoital orgasms on menstrual days. By contrast, the wives did not experience any increased sexual frustration during menstruation. The heterosexual non-intercourse-related orgasm rate among these women was relatively stable throughout their cycle. Morris and Udry suggested that the different patterns of desire levels for husbands and wives may have a biological base and that the behavioral patterns observed in their study represent a social adjustment to this difference.

The level of estrogen and progesterone (hormones secreted by the ovaries) is lower during menstruation, which may play a role in decreased sexual desire. The lowered hormone levels may also reduce vaginal lubrication. These two factors may combine to decrease a woman's sexual enjoyment during menstruation. It's likely that additional factors also play a role in sexuality in relation to the menstrual cycle. Many women, however, don't experience any differences in their sexual desire or activity across their menstrual cycle. Some women even find it easier to express their sexuality and to experience orgasms during menstruation, perhaps because they know their chance of pregnancy is lower (although it's not zero) than at other times of the month.

Is a woman more likely to become pregnant if she has an orgasm?

POSSIBLY. ONE EFFECT OF orgasm is to increase a suction produced by wave-like contractions of the uterus. During orgasm in sexual intercourse, suction draws ejaculated semen that is deposited near the cervix into the uterus. When a woman experiences orgasm, the hormone oxytocin is released into the bloodstream by the pituitary gland. The oxytocin then stimulates the muscles of the uterus, which contract more forcefully and increase the amount of suction. With female orgasm, more semen (and so more sperm) enters the uterus, where it is then pulled more toward the left or right side, depending on whether the left or right ovary will release a mature egg (ovum) during that particular menstrual cycle.

Further evidence of the effect of orgasm on pregnancy is a report that women whose orgasm occurs just *after* their partner ejaculates retain more semen (and so more sperm) in their vagina than women whose orgasm occurs just *before* their partner ejaculates. The study authors speculated that, by increasing the suction action of the uterus, a woman's orgasm can increase the retention of sperm in the vagina, which could make more sperm available for fertilizing an egg. Some valid criticisms have been made of the methods used in these experiments, but there is still good evidence to suggest that a woman's orgasm may increase the chance of pregnancy.

Is it safe to have orgasms during pregnancy?

THERE IS CONTROVERSY AMONG researchers about whether or not intercourse during pregnancy affects (causes or prevents) premature delivery. One scientific report, published in 2001, found that intercourse during the "last few weeks of pregnancy appears to increase the risk of preterm delivery." The study supported an earlier claim by researchers who stated that the male-on-top position was associated with premature rupture of the membranes. However, other researchers have concluded that intercourse during late pregnancy is associated with a *reduced* risk of preterm delivery. Yet another study found that intercourse earlier in pregnancy was not associated with an increased risk of preterm delivery (although intercourse during pregnancy *was* associated with an increased incidence of preterm delivery in women with a lower genital tract infection). So, given all these contradictory findings, couples should consult with their physician for individualized advice on the safety of intercourse during pregnancy.

On a different but related topic: many women worry that sexual activity and orgasm during pregnancy could harm the fetus. In addition to the possible risks associated with preterm delivery mentioned above, there is a risk to the fetus if the woman acquires a sexually transmitted infection, so safer sex practices are advisable.

Does childbirth affect orgasm?

YES, ORGASM CAN BE affected in a variety of ways by childbirth. The birth process itself has been described as orgasmic. In a 2007 interview study of eleven women, Danielle Harel characterized two types of sexual experience during childbirth as described by these women: "Unexpected birthgasms were described as surprising orgasms while pushing out or delivering the baby . . . They occurred without any sexual stimulation or use of fantasy, and were not perceived by the women in this sample as erotic or 'sexual' in nature . . . Passionate birth was experienced by the women in the sample who chose to incorporate their sexuality openly and intentionally in the birth process, and who allowed themselves to fully explore it. They made love, vocalized, kissed passionately, and some of them masturbated to ease the pain."

A different facet of the effect of childbirth involves its effect on the sexual interaction between the parents. Researcher Kirsten von Sydow analyzed fifty-nine research articles published between 1959 and 1996 that were related to parents' sexual function and behavior during pregnancy and up to six months after the birth of their child. On average, female sexual interest and frequency of intercourse decline slightly in the first trimester of pregnancy and decrease sharply in the third trimester. Many couples don't have intercourse during the two months or so before the due date. After delivery, sexual interest and activity tend to be diminished for several months compared with pre-pregnancy levels, and sexual problems are common. However, not all couples follow this pattern. Sexual responsiveness and capacity to experience orgasm differ from one couple to another.

When a child is born, the mother undergoes major emotional, psychological, and physiological changes, especially if she is a first-time mother. At the same time, the father undergoes major emotional changes of his own. Changing roles within the relationship can bring the couple closer or drive them apart. The mother and the father, having adjusted to each other as independent adults, now must direct their attention to, and become responsible for, a newborn dependent being. The prior dual relationship, which may have involved a strong sexual bond and sharing the experience of orgasm, suddenly becomes a triangular relationship.

A simple lack of information about sexual relations and orgasms during and after pregnancy could affect a couple's relationship after childbirth. For example, the couple might abstain from sexual intercourse if they are unsure of the risk of infection or, in the case of a caesarian delivery, they worry about rupturing the stitches. A woman may experience a decline in sexual interest and activity in the period after delivery (the "postpartum" period) for many reasons, including the physical effects of breastfeeding, vaginal delivery, surgical vaginal delivery (in more complicated births), instrument delivery (use of vacuum extraction or forceps to help deliver the baby), trauma to the perineum (the skin between the vagina and anus), vaginal tearing, and episiotomy (a surgical incision made in the perineum during childbirth). Vaginal delivery can reduce the strength of the pelvic floor muscles, although studies have not shown that this adversely affects a woman's sexual functioning. Nevertheless, some women do find that starting Kegel exercises before and after childbirth can restore their strength and can empower a woman who wants to resume her prior level of sexual activity.

Most women say that the main reasons for not having an active sex life for at least a few weeks after childbirth are simply physical exhaustion from the birth, lack of sleep, and adjusting to the changed lifestyle with the new bundle of joy. It's important to reinstate sexual life *gradually* after childbirth. Some of the major organs of a woman's body are involved in the process of childbirth. After a painful vaginal birth, a woman may associate the vagina with pain rather than with pleasure. A new mother may need time to reintroduce her vagina to pleasurable sensations. Nipples and breasts, perhaps once thought of as part of the sexual relationship, now take on a new purpose.

The reactions of the father can have an important impact on the mother's interest in resuming the couple's sexual relationship. Physical affection, not necessarily genital or even sexual, can help reestablish a man's intimate relationship with the new mother. The new father should reassure the new mother about her bodily changes after pregnancy and birth and should appreciate that it will take time for her to become ready, physically and emotionally, to resume her sexual life.

How do hormones affect women's orgasms?

HORMONES ARE SECRETED BY the endocrine glands, which include the gonads (ovaries and testicles), adrenals, pituitary, thyroid, and pancreas. The gonads are directly involved in the development and control of sexual behavior through the secretion of their hormones: estrogens, androgens (including testosterone), and progestogens (including progesterone).

There is a general belief that sexual activity, including orgasm, is strongly influenced by hormones. So it's logical to expect that taking hormones, for any reason, will affect orgasm and other components of sexual behavior. This turns out to be sometimes true, sometimes not, depending on the hormone and the preexisting levels of that hormone in the body.

Surprisingly, testosterone, which is commonly thought of as the "male hormone," is actually the hormone that is most closely related to the expression of sexual response in women. A large number of carefully controlled studies have recently shown that the application of a transdermal androgen patch—designed to release low amounts of testosterone through the skin (transdermally) and into the bloodstream—has positive effects on all components of women's sexual response, including orgasm and sexual satisfaction. This is found to occur for postmenopausal women, women who have had their ovaries removed, and women who have an androgen-insufficiency disorder. These treatments are designed to provide women with amounts of testosterone that are high enough to mimic the normal levels produced by the ovaries (and by the adrenals), but low enough to avoid unwanted (masculinizing) side effects.

Recently, a synthetic steroid known as tibolone (which has estrogenic, progestogenic, and androgenic effects) has been introduced in Europe and other countries, but not in the United States, for the treatment of sexual disorders in women. Results coming from different institutions indicate that this synthetic hormone effectively improves most aspects of sexual response, including orgasm. Tibolone has been associated with a slightly increased risk of stroke.

Another use of hormones, of course, by millions of women worldwide, is as a method of contraception. Oral contraceptives use a combination of estrogens and progestins (synthetic progestogens). Reports on the effects of these contraceptives on sexual response are extremely variable—a small percentage of women complain of negative effects, and a similarly small percentage report a positive effect. In most cases, studies show that these effects are not significantly different from those obtained with a placebo (an intentionally inactive pill that is identical in outward appearance to the active pill containing the hormones).

Three

Men's Orgasms

How does a penis become erect?

SEXUAL STIMULATION OF THE penis or psychogenic (cognitively in-duced) arousal activates specialized nerves that travel from the pelvic region of the spinal cord to the penis. These nerves release nitric oxide (NO) and other nerve products (neurotransmitters) that relax the smooth muscles and blood vessels of the penis (*smooth* describes muscles that, unlike skeletal muscles, are not under our voluntary control). Relaxation of these muscles allows increased blood flow into the penis. Spongy tissues (the corpora cavernosa) in the penis become filled (en-gorged) with blood and expand rapidly. There is a capsule (the tunica albuginea) that surrounds the internal penile tissues, which is made of connective tissue and is flexible but not stretchable. When the corpora cavernosa become engorged with blood, they "inflate" against the cap-sule, making the penis rigid. The compression inside the penis almost totally closes down the veins that drain blood from the penis, so blood is trapped in the penile tissues, maintaining the erection.

Because erection is so dependent on an adequate blood flow, the con-dition known as erectile dysfunction can provide an early warning sign,

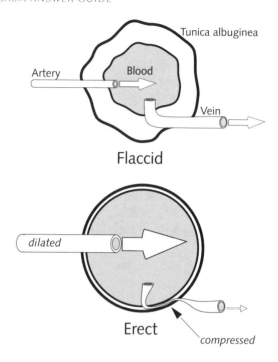

Penile erection. Erection occurs as a result of a two-stage process. The top diagram shows (in cross section) the penis before erection. In the first stage of erection, the arteries that supply the penis dilate, allowing more blood to enter and fill the open spaces ("sinuses") of the penis The amount of inflation is limited by a flexible but non-expandable membrane (like a mylar balloon), the tunica albuginea, which envelops the penile tissues. In the second stage of erection, the veins that drain blood from the penis get squeezed almost shut against the tunica albuginea. The resulting pressurized accumulation of blood in the penis produces the erection.

or red flag, for impending vascular (blood vessel) disease. Erectile dysfunction in men who have no other symptoms of vascular disease may be a marker of a "silent" vascular disorder, especially coronary artery disease, and this has become an important new means of identifying men at risk for such disease.

How do men ejaculate?

Ejaculation requires precise coordination among several different organs, from the testicles to the penis. Two intriguing aspects of ejaculation are: First, how exactly are the spurts of semen produced? Second, is the pleasurable sensation of orgasm a consequence of the sensory activity produced by the mechanics of ejaculation, or is it mainly a brain phenomenon that is pleasantly enhanced by the sensory activity generated by the expulsive flow of semen at ejaculation? This is a case in which understanding the structure of a system is key to understanding its function.

From a purely mechanical standpoint, contraction of the muscles of the male genital system is, by itself, not strong enough or sudden enough to account for the emission of semen in spurts. Instead, the spurts are produced by precise timing between muscle contractions of the ejaculatory duct system and the sphincter muscles (valves that act much like purse strings) situated in the path of the semen flow. In sequence, this is what happens: (1) the ducts fill with semen (the process of "emission"); (2) pressure builds up behind a closed sphincter valve (the semen-filled duct and the sphincter together are aptly called the "pressure chamber"); (3) a sudden release of the sphincter valve emits a spurt of semen ("ejaculation"); (4) the ejaculatory ducts fill up again behind the re-closed sphincter; and (5) a repeat of the process results in another spurt of semen. This sequence of events repeats several times in rapid succession in a matter of a few seconds.

The initial, emission, stage in the ejaculation process is produced by contractions of the muscles in several places: in the capsules of the testicles, seminal vesicles, and prostate, and in the ducts of the epididymis and vas deferens. The vas deferens contracts as a unit, from one end (at the caudal, or tail-end, epididymis) to the other (at the ejaculatory duct of the prostate); the seminal vesicles contract by peristalsis (traveling waves of muscle contraction and relaxation that propel the semen through this tubular organ).

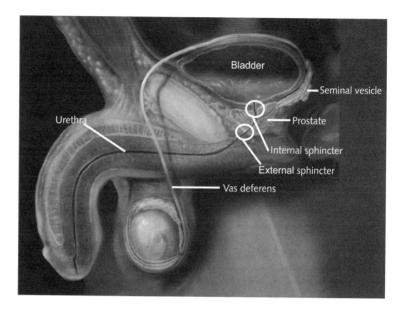

The path taken by sperm during ejaculation. Sperm travel from the testicles through the vas deferens (one on each side) to exit the body through the urethra. The seminal vesicles and prostate contribute the seminal fluid that carries and nourishes the sperm. The external and internal sphincters consist of rings of muscle that surround and squeeze shut the urethra. Contractions of the vas deferens tubes and the seminal vesicles during sexual stimulation, building up to ejaculation, increase the pressure against the closed sphincters. At orgasm, the external sphincter relaxes rhythmically, enabling the pressurized semen to be released in spurts. (Image courtesy Alexander Tsiaras, TheVisualMD.com)

Contraction of the internal sphincter prevents the backflow of semen into the bladder. If this sphincter fails to close sufficiently during ejaculation, semen can make a U turn and enter the urinary bladder, a process known as "retrograde ejaculation."

At orgasm, under the control of the pudendal nerves, the pelvic muscles start contracting rhythmically and involuntarily. A sphincter opens and closes in closely coordinated timing with the contraction of specific muscles. The intermittent opening and closing aids in propulsion of the semen through the urethra. Studies have shown the importance of the coordination of the opening and closing of this sphincter. If the sphincter becomes paralyzed or is incapacitated by experimental anesthesia, a dripping seminal emission, rather than ejaculation, occurs.

Does a penis need to be hard to have an orgasm?

GILES BRINDLEY NOTED IN 1983 that ejaculation and orgasm don't necessarily require erection. In Brindley's studies, men were equipped with a mechanical clamp that squeezed shut the pudendal arteries—the arteries that supply blood to the penis. The men were still able to ejaculate and experience orgasm, even though the penis remained entirely flaccid (non-erect). In other words, the nerves that convey sensations from the penis during stimulation do so whether the penis is erect or flaccid. Many men who have had surgery for prostate cancer are able to experience orgasm without erection (men with successful nerve-sparing prostate surgery will most likely continue to have erections).

Why is the penis so sensitive after an orgasm?

SOME MEN EXPERIENCE GREATLY increased sensitivity (hypersensitivity), and even pain, of the penis after orgasm. The physiological basis for this hypersensitivity is not known. During penetrative sex, the friction of the skin of the penis against the walls of the vagina (or other surface) could make the skin sensitive. There is some evidence that release of the hormone prolactin into the bloodstream at orgasm may increase the sensitivity of the penis, as well as the nipples.

There is no consensus among researchers as to whether circumcision at infancy affects the sensitivity of the penis. Abnormally low penile sensitivity, as a result of trauma to the genital region, injury to the penile sensory (pudendal) nerves, or diabetes, can result in erectile dysfunction.

Can a man have an orgasm without stimulation of his penis?

YES, MOST MEN HAVE experienced orgasm without obvious penile stimulation, while asleep (commonly known as wet dreams, or more technically as nocturnal emissions). In rare cases, men have reported experiencing orgasm without mechanical (e.g., tactile) stimulation while fully awake. According to an extensive study by Kinsey and his colleagues in 1948, three or four men in five thousand claimed to have experienced ejaculatory orgasm without mechanical stimulation while awake. Some men who practice a specialized form of forced rapid deep breathing combined with Tantric meditation ("fire breath") claim that they experience orgasms in the absence of physical genital stimulation.

Can men experience ejaculation without orgasm, or orgasm without ejaculation?

YES, MEN CAN EXPERIENCE orgasm with no ejaculatory fluid expelled, and they can ejaculate without feeling the pleasure of orgasm.

There are certain conditions that prevent ejaculation despite an erection and orgasm. These include surgery affecting the genital system, such as prostatectomy (removal of the prostate gland, typically as a treatment for cancer); certain psychiatric conditions, such as obsessive compulsive disorder (for example, when a man is overly concerned about hygiene and thinks ejaculation will be messy); psychological/psychosexual issues, such as fear of impregnating a partner, fear of losing control, or cultural inhibitions; and side effects of certain medications such as SSRIs (selective serotonin reuptake inhibitors), which are prescribed as antidepressants (for example, citalopram or fluoxetine). Although SSRIs and other medications can interfere with sexual desire and function, individuals should not discontinue these medications without consulting their physician, because serious complications could result. Interference with ejaculation may also result from a progressive neurological disease such as MS (multiple sclerosis), from neurological damage resulting from stroke or spinal cord injury, or from hormonal deficiencies.

By contrast, there are some conditions in which a man can ejaculate in the absence of erection or orgasm. These include severe cases of premature ejaculation (early ejaculation), in which the man ejaculates before developing an erection or before physical stimulation of the penis; psychological factors, such as overexcitement, fear of intimacy, or relationship issues; psychiatric disorders such as severe schizophrenia; complications after surgery involving the genital system; and other conditions such as hormone imbalance, progressive neurological disorders, chronic diabetes, abuse of drugs or alcohol, and brain or spinal cord injury.

Some men voluntarily separate their orgasm from ejaculation. They do so by noting the point after which they can't hold back (the point of "ejaculatory inevitability") and training themselves to control their ejaculation just before reaching this point. By delaying ejaculation in this way, they claim to experience an enjoyable, prolonged sexual session with their partner, with a deeper and more intense sexual intimacy. An example of this practice is the teaching of Tantric sex, through which a man learns to be orgasmic while delaying ejaculation until he feels ready.

Why do some men become so sleepy after an orgasm?

NOBODY KNOWS FOR SURE. However, sleepiness in men after orgasm is very common. The physical exertion of sexual intercourse can feel as if it's considerable, but a 175-pound man participating in vigorous sex for thirty minutes expends only 63 calories. If he had spent the same amount of time jogging, he would have used 288 calories (and most joggers claim to feel energized, not sleepy, after their run). So, it's probably something other than physical exertion that accounts for the sleepy feeling after orgasm. We do know that women seem to feel less tired than men after orgasm. Men share their tendency to want to doze with at least one other mammal. Carefully constructed laboratory studies showed that male rats fall deeply asleep shortly after mating (but, so do female rabbits!).

In one study, of five men and five women, researchers compared three conditions: masturbation to orgasm with a latency of about fifteen minutes; masturbation for fifteen minutes, while intentionally refraining from orgasm; and reading a newspaper for fifteen minutes. They found no significant difference among the three conditions in the time delay between the event and when the person fell asleep, or in the duration of sleep, or in the type of sleep pattern. However, this study was just a start, not an ideal way to study this topic. Many disruptive factors could account for the lack of difference among the three conditions in the study, including the laboratory setting, the fact that an investigator entered the room after every fifteen-minute period to remove the anal probe used to measure orgasmic muscular contractions, the presence of EEG (electroencephalogram) electrodes to measure sleep, the possible sleep-inducing effect of reading a newspaper, the combining of the data for the men and the women, and the absence of the personal physical and emotional interactions inherent in sexual encounters. So, with our present state of knowledge about any connection between orgasm and sleep, anecdotal reports, jokes, and cartoons appear to characterize reality better than does the existing scientific research!

Still, even though science has yet to offer a satisfactory explanation for the widely reported tendency of men (and some women) to become sleepy after orgasm, at least knowing that this sleepiness is so common offers some comfort to those who may "take it personally." As humans, many of us have the capacity to generate a modicum of conversation and hugging and caressing in the aftermath of orgasm, at least for a while. To our male readers, especially, we suggest giving it a try. An interlude of post-orgasm tender bonding—even if only briefly, before sleep overwhelms—doesn't hurt.

What is the clear fluid that comes out of the penis before ejaculation?

SECRETION OF THIS PRE-EJACULATORY fluid, which in some cases starts during sexual foreplay, can be surprisingly abundant—half to one milliliter (1 mL is about one-fifth of a teaspoonful). The presence of this fluid is evidence of a high level of sexual arousal. For many years it was associated with voluptuous thinking, and medieval writers called it "the distillate of love."

Long before the nineteenth century, when William Cowper described the glands involved in this secretion, the secreted fluid was recognized as being different from semen. There is now good evidence that the secretion comes from a small set of structures named Cowper's glands, in honor of their discoverer (and also called the bulbo-urethral glands). Cowper's glands, together with the prostate and seminal vesicles, comprise the "sex accessory" glands in men. Cowper's glands are the male counterpart of women's Bartholin's glands (or greater vestibular glands), which produce some of the vaginal fluid.

The secretion from Cowper's glands is composed of a clear fluid with a high concentration of glycoproteins (proteins with some sugars attached). The fluid neutralizes the acidity of the urine residue in the man's urethra and the normal acidity of the vaginal environment. It may also provide lubrication for the penis during intercourse. For some time it was thought that this secretion could contain some stray sperm that escape from the epididymis before ejaculation, and that this could explain unexpected pregnancies during coitus interruptus (a contraceptive technique in which the man withdraws his penis from the vagina before ejaculating). However, recent studies have shown that the pre-ejaculatory fluid that leaks from the tip of the penis during sexual stimulation does not contain any sperm.

What is the difference between semen and sperm?

SEMEN (ALSO CALLED SEMINAL fluid, seminal plasma, or ejaculatory fluid) consists of a combination of secretions from the testicles, epididymis, vas deferens, seminal vesicles, prostate, and Cowper's glands.

When the free-swimming sperm cells (also called spermatozoa) leave the testicles (where they are produced), they enter, on each side, a long, convoluted tube—the epididymis—situated above the testicles. The sperm are mixed with a fluid secreted by the epididymis and testicles, and this mixture moves slowly toward the vas deferens, a slightly wider tube than the epididymis. (The paired vas deferens tubes, left and right, are the tubes that are "tied" in the vasectomy procedure.) After passing through the vas deferens on each side, the sperm and fluids enter the urethra, the tube that also transports urine from the bladder. During this journey, the sperm acquire their capacity to fertilize the ovum (a process termed "capacitation"). This involves a series of physical and chemical changes in the "head" of the sperm (the acrosome, as distinct from the sperm's moving tail). The semen is therefore a mixture of various fluids; it conveys the sperm.

The fluids that comprise semen serve a variety of functions. They provide for more powerful ejaculation and contain a source of energy for the vigorously swimming sperm, in the form of fructose (a sugar) and inositol (another type of nutrient). The semen also contains prostaglandins (secreted by the prostate gland), which stimulate contraction of the muscles of the female reproductive tract, assisting the sperm in their voyage toward the egg (ovum).

The normal color of ejaculatory fluid is a semitransparent yellowish color. If any major changes occur in the color or texture of ejaculatory fluid (for example, becoming orange, thick and white, or with drops of blood), it's advisable for a man to consult his physician. A physician should always be alerted if ejaculation is combined with a feeling of urgency to urinate, a burning sensation when urinating, or pain, because these may be signs of a urinary tract infection or an STI (sexually transmitted infection), which, if untreated, could lead to kidney damage or other serious complications.

Why does semen change from opaque to transparent?

EJACULATED HUMAN SEMEN TYPICALLY appears opaque—a grayish-white mass mixed with a clear liquid. The mass consists of protein that is coagulated (jelled) by an enzyme secreted by the seminal vesicles. The clear liquid is secreted mainly by the prostate gland and Cowper's glands.

Within about ten to twenty minutes of ejaculation, the opaque mass begins to change into a clear liquid. This change is due to the action of another enzyme, known as seminin, that is secreted into the semen by the prostate gland. This enzyme gives a characteristic aroma to the semen. As an aside, "seminin" is another name for "prostate-specific antigen," or PSA. The level of PSA in the bloodstream is commonly used to screen for prostate cancer. The normal function of PSA—or seminin—is to liberate the sperm from the coagulated semen so that the sperm cells are free to move toward the egg.

Evidence suggests that the coagulated mass in semen restricts the free movement of the ejaculated sperm, which probably has the effect of "herding" them, keeping them near the cervix, which is the gateway to the uterus. Thus the semen helps keep the sperm from flowing out of the vagina. Then, seminin starts to convert the coagulated mass into a clear liquid (a process called liquefaction), allowing the sperm to swim out of the mass and enter the uterus on their way to the egg.

This coagulation function of semen is developed to an extreme in some rodents. In these animals, coagulation forms a "copulatory plug" almost instantaneously after ejaculation into the vagina. The copulatory plug has the texture of dried rubber cement. It forms a hard piston that fills the inner end of the vagina just in front of the cervix, trapping the sperm, under pressure, between the tip of the plug and the cervix. The pressure forces the semen and sperm through the cervix and into the uterus.

What causes differences in the amount and characteristics of semen ejaculated?

THE PROCESS OF EJACULATION in men has been investigated by numerous techniques, including genital physiological recordings, genital imaging, and brain imaging. Several genital organs contribute to semen. A typical orgasm produces about five milliliters (5 mL; about one teaspoonful) of semen, which has the following components: sperm cells and secretions from the seminal vesicles (3 mL), prostate (1.5 to 2 mL), Cowper's glands (0.5 mL), and glands of Littre, also known as preputial glands (0.1 to 0.2 mL). The amount, aroma, taste, texture, density, and color of semen vary from person to person and from time to time in each individual. Temperature, physical activity, diet, and recent ejaculations can also affect the properties and amount of the fluid. In the case of two closely successive ejaculations, the second volume is typically less than the first.

How do hormones affect men's orgasms?

MEN'S SEXUAL BEHAVIOR AND sexual function, including orgasm, are influenced by the action of hormones. A man's natural steroid hormones, in particular, affect sexual processes. These hormones are secreted into the bloodstream by the gonads (testicles) and by the adrenal glands (specifically, the part of the gland known as the adrenal cortex). The term *steroid* refers to their chemical structure, and this family of chemicals includes the sex steroids (androgens, estrogens, and progestins) and the corticoids (which are secreted by the adrenal cortex). By far the most important male hormone is testosterone, an androgen, which is secreted almost exclusively by the testicles. Castrating males (surgically removing the testicles) greatly affects their sexual functioning.

Castration has been carried out in men and animals since prehistoric times. It's a relatively easy operation, because of the accessibility of the testicles, and was practiced by several cultures for its biological and psychological effects. In the middle of the nineteenth century, it was observed that castration of roosters not only induced physical changes but also inhibited their sexual behavior. Early scientists found that the effects of castration could be reversed when a testicular graft was placed into the castrated rooster. This type of experiment has been repeated in many mammalian species, including humans, with the same results. Indeed, the rooster experiment is credited with creating the entire field of endocrinology (the study of hormones and their effects). Despite these known effects of drastically reducing testosterone levels by castration, normal levels of testosterone do not guarantee normal sexual behavior and orgasm.

It isn't always possible to establish a clear correlation between levels of testosterone circulating in the bloodstream and sexual activity (desire, arousability, and orgasm), but we do know that a clear and abrupt decrease in sexual interest may occur in healthy men when treated with drugs that inhibit their testosterone secretion.

We also know that medical treatment with testosterone affects orgasms. In men, aging is often associated with a lowered secretion of testosterone, and sexual disorders including anorgasmia (inability to have an orgasm) can occur. According to a recent study, 30 percent of men over the age of sixty have clear signs of what is known as hypogonadism (low levels of androgen secretion). Currently, testosterone is the usual treatment for these men, and most studies indicate a clear improvement in sexual life following administration of the hormone. Injections of a long-acting chemical derivative of testosterone (testosterone undecanoate) have often been used successfully to improve men's sexual activity and ability to experience orgasm. In more recent studies, testosterone has been administered transdermally (through the skin), by a skin patch that delivers constant, low amounts of the hormone into the bloodstream. Although there is no doubt that testosterone improves sexual life in hypogonadal men, it's not clear how it works, whether through its action on brain structures related to sexual desire and orgasm or, indirectly, by increasing physical energy and/or by maintaining the genital structures.

There has been some controversy about the side effects of testosterone treatments for men with hypogonadism. Some researchers worry, for example, that the treatments might activate dormant prostate cancer in older men or might cause immunodeficiency. In the United States, a controversy between the Endocrine Society and a National Institutes of Health panel occurred only a few years ago on this topic. In recent well-controlled studies using the dosages actually used for treatment of hypogonadism, no serious side effects occurred. Indeed, positive effects on cardiovascular health were reported when proper doses of testosterone were administered. However, most physicians are not likely to prescribe testosterone for men who have undergone treatment for prostate cancer.

There is no consensus on whether testosterone can act as an aphrodisiac. Some studies have reported that testosterone administered to men with normal levels of testosterone can increase sexual enjoyment and activity. However, other studies suggest there is no benefit to increasing the androgen level beyond that of normal secretions by the testicles.

At the other extreme, treatment with certain steroids has been used to *inhibit* undesired male sexual behavior, such as pedophilia (sex with children), with variable success. For example, a synthetic progestin (medroxy-progesterone) has been reported to inhibit undesired sexual behavior. It acts by inhibiting the secretion of the pituitary hormones that maintain the production of testosterone by the testicles. Another way to decrease unwanted sexual activity is by the use of drugs known as anti-androgens (such as cyproterone acetate), which don't affect testosterone secretion but instead prevent the action of the hormone in the brain, by preventing its interaction with specific receptors in brain neurons and other cells.

In yet another use of steroids, for more than thirty years, men of all ages have been using anabolic steroids (androgens that stimulate protein synthesis, particularly in muscle) for bodybuilding. One of these steroids is 5-alpha-dihydrotestosterone (DHT), which is a normal metabolic product of testosterone. In most experimental animals, anabolic steroids such as DHT are much less potent in stimulating sexual behavior than is testosterone, and apparently the same is true in men. Some recent studies, however, indicate that when administered together with estrogen, DHT can be used to treat male anorgasmia and several other types of sexual disorder.

Four

Hows and Whys of Orgasm

How do legal and illegal drugs affect orgasm?

A LARGE VARIETY OF DRUGS are known to affect orgasm in positive or negative ways. In many cases, the reports of positive effects are anecdotal or have been described in uncontrolled (that is, not scientifically rigorous) studies using a small number of individuals. So we need to take some claims about the positive effects of certain drugs with a grain of salt. However, there is reliable information, based on sound scientific studies, about the effect on orgasm of several drugs, particularly prescription drugs that are used to treat sexually and non-sexually related health problems. We will do our best to explain what is known about the effects of many drugs, legal and illegal, on orgasm. It's important to keep in mind that a lot of drugs can have serious side effects and their use should not be considered lightly.

The positive effect of steroids, particularly testosterone, on orgasm in both men and women has been established in many well-controlled studies. Testosterone is found to be effective for individuals with low levels of testosterone in their bloodstream, usually older men or post-menopausal women. Its possible aphrodisiac effect on individuals who have normal levels of steroids produced by their gonads (testicles and ovaries) remains controversial.

Yohimbine has for many years had the reputation of being an aphrodisiac, and this has been validated in several studies. This drug counteracts several aspects of sexual disorders. Initially, yohimbine was used to facilitate or prolong penile erection, but it was later found to improve sexual arousal and orgasm as well. It acts mainly by increasing the release of noradrenaline (also called norepinephrine), a neurotransmitter in the brain and nerves that is involved in various aspects of sexual activity.

We need to get a bit technical here to explain how yohimbine works, but this information is also useful in understanding the actions of some other drugs. Neurons (nerve cells) that produce noradrenaline have a particular type of receptor, called an "autoreceptor," that recognizes and responds specifically to the same neurotransmitter that the cell produces. In this case, neurons that produce and dispense noradrenaline contain autoreceptors (called alpha-2 receptors) on their surface that respond to their own or other neurons' released noradrenaline by slowing down the further release of their own noradenaline. This is a process called "negative feedback." It's similar to how a thermostat works, responding to the increased temperature in the room by turning off the source of heat—the furnace. Yohimbine has its effect by blocking the action of noradrenaline on the neuron's autoreceptor (much like a key that breaks off in a lock so that another key can't be inserted into the lock). This results in the continued release of noradrenaline from the neuron, and this increased noradrenaline has an orgasm-stimulating effect. Again using the analogy of the thermostat, it's as if the thermostat is blocked from sensing when the room gets warm, so it fails to shut off the furnace, and the room gets hotter.

Yohimbine is effective when taken two to four hours before sexual activity. An effective dose of yohimbine to counteract orgasmic dysfunction in men is about twenty milligrams. At this dose, side effects seem minor. There is insufficient comparable information for women.

Another neurotransmitter that has a stimulating effect on orgasm is dopamine. Drugs such as amphetamine that stimulate the release of dopamine can stimulate or prolong orgasm. However, the undesirable side effects of amphetamine, particularly serious paranoid schizophrenic symptoms, prevent its medical use for the treatment of sexual disorders.

Cocaine has a similar effect of increasing the levels of dopamine in specific brain regions, thereby stimulating orgasm in men and women. Cocaine blocks the reabsorption (reuptake) of dopamine by the neurons that released it, keeping it available to neighboring neurons—which increases the stimulatory effect of the dopamine. Because cocaine is highly addictive, its use as a treatment for sexual disorders is not recommended.

The antidepressant drugs known as selective serotonin reuptake inhibitors (SSRIs) have a negative effect on orgasm and other sexual functions. Since the nineteenth century, depression has been known to be associated with sexual disorders, and it was logical to think that an improvement in the depressive illness would result in improvement of sexual function. So, it's ironic that a class of drugs that reduces the effects of depression creates sexual disorders as a side effect. Recent studies suggest that 90 percent of patients taking antidepressants that increase serotonin levels—which is how SSRIs work—experience sexual disorders. The SSRIs act by interfering with the reuptake of serotonin into the serotonin-producing neurons, thereby prolonging the action of serotonin on neighboring neurons. Some recent studies that examine specific aspects of sexual disorders in patients treated for major depression with SSRIs and other medications show that men are more likely than women to have problems experiencing orgasms.

The first effective antidepressants introduced into clinical practice were the MAO inhibitors (monoamine oxidase inhibitors). Monoamine oxidase is an enzyme that breaks down and inactivates the class of neurotransmitters known as the monoamines. These include noradrenaline, dopamine, and serotonin. By inhibiting this breakdown, MAO inhibitors increase the levels of these three monoamines in the brain. Although dopamine and noradrenaline, as we've seen, tend to stimulate orgasm, these effects are counteracted by the increased levels of serotonin, which has an overriding inhibitory effect on sexual responses.

Fortunately, several new antidepressant drugs avoid the side effect of sexual disorders, and some of them even enhance sexual responses. Studies show particularly consistent results in enhancing orgasm with the use of bupropion. In addition, a new generation of antidepressants, such as moclobemide, which are known as "reversible inhibitors of MAO," are reported to strongly stimulate orgasm in some individuals.

Another class of frequently prescribed drugs that depress sexual activity is the antipsychotics, which are used for treating schizophrenia and a particular form of depression known as malignant depression. These were among the first drugs that were recognized to impair or prevent orgasm in men and women.

More recent, "atypical" antipsychotics such as clozapine, which act on several types of neurotransmitter receptors other than the dopamine receptor, apparently have a less negative effect on orgasm and sexual activity than other antipsychotics.

There is a widespread belief that certain recreational stimulant drugs enhance or alter sexual pleasure and orgasm. Many marijuana users claim they have more prolonged, intense, and hence more rewarding orgasms than those experienced without the drug. These marijuana-related changes in the quality of orgasm, rather than changes in frequency or in ease of stimulation, are difficult to evaluate. Some well-controlled studies do report an increase in awareness of muscular contractions in the genital area during orgasm. Perhaps it's more significant, however, that a recent analysis of sexual disorders resulting from drug use in 3,004 men and women found that chronic use of marijuana was significantly associated with anorgasmia.

The drug Ecstasy, a derivative of amphetamine, is considered to affect social interactions and sexual response. Some studies were designed to test the reported aphrodisiac effects of this drug. Sexual desire was increased in most men and women taking Ecstasy, although, paradoxically, erectile dysfunction was noted in 40 percent of the men. Some Ecstasy users claim to experience a different, more rewarding type of orgasm, but this effect is difficult to evaluate objectively.

A variety of drugs that have the common property of depressing the central nervous system (brain and spinal cord), including alcohol, opiates, barbiturates, and benzodiazepines (such as diazepam), have at times been described as reducing social inhibitions to sexual intercourse. In some cases, when sexual activity is inhibited by high levels of anxiety, moderate amounts of alcohol or diazepam are found to facilitate sexual activity, but in general these drugs impair orgasm.

Why do people sometimes experience orgasms while asleep?

Unfortunately, there is very limited scientific research on orgasms while sleeping. One question that is raised is whether the person experiencing the orgasm was in fact making contact between his or her genitals and the bed or sheets. However, there is good reason to believe that orgasms while sleeping are not, in fact, the result of genital stimulation but instead are created in the brain. For example, men and women with spinal cord injuries—with no nerve connections between their external genitals and their brain—are known to experience orgasms while asleep.

In a rare, and lucky, case in a laboratory study, researchers made physiological measurements while a woman had an orgasm during a dream. When she awoke, the woman described the dream and the orgasm she had experienced. The researchers reported that the rate of blood flow to her vagina, her heart rate, and her respiration rate all increased during the dream. Specifically, her heart rate increased from 50 to 100 beats per minute, her respiration rate increased from 12 to 22 breaths per minute, and she had a "very marked" increase in vaginal blood flow. Her vagina showed cyclic episodes of engorgement with blood during her REM (rapid eye movement) sleep stages. In sleep studies, the greater ease of measuring penile erection than vaginal blood flow has resulted in research showing that men typically have penile engorgement during 95 percent of REM sleep stages.

It is likely, based on all these observations and other, less scientific reports, that orgasms during sleep are not a response to genital stimulation, but rather are the result of brain activity. In other words, the physiological responses seem not to be "reflexive" responses to genital stimulation but to be generated intrinsically by the brain. So, it seems that during sleep, the brain can behave in a way that turns on all the systems involved in the experience of orgasm.

Why do people say that orgasms happen in the brain?

THE ANSWER DEPENDS LARGELY on what we mean by "happens." Everything a person feels is sensed in the brain. So, orgasms are *felt* in the brain, and to some that means they *happen* in the brain. But the process of orgasm involves virtually every body system. Looked at in this way, the brain is not the only place where orgasms "happen," but rather, the brain is the conductor of the orgasmic orchestra.

In recent years, technology has made it possible to directly observe three-dimensional activity in the human brain. This has led to an explosion of research that correlates activity in specific brain regions with people's perceptions and feelings. Some investigators have begun to analyze the parts of the brain that are activated by genital stimulation and orgasm, through the use of a technology called "functional magnetic resonance imaging," or functional MRI, or simply fMRI. All the major regions of the brain become activated during orgasm. Perhaps this is not surprising, because many different body systems are activated during orgasm—systems that are under the influence of the brain. The muscles of the arms, legs, trunk, face, and genitals become more active, as do the muscles that produce increased heart rate, blood pressure, uterine contractions, and dilation of the pupils. Sweating and

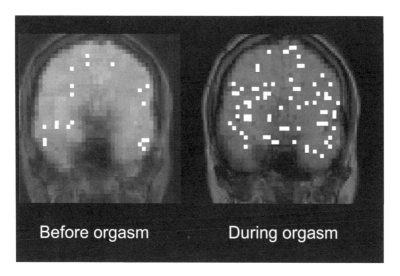

Before orgasm   During orgasm

Images of brain activity recorded by fMRI (functional magnetic resonance imaging). The left image is of a woman's brain during the first minute of vaginal self-stimulation. The image on the right shows the same brain several minutes later, during orgasm. The much greater brain activity during orgasm is revealed by the regions covered with white squares.

the secretion of hormones (including oxytocin and prolactin) increase, while arousal and pleasurable feelings intensify. Using fMRI, researchers can visualize these events in the brain. If you compare the fMRIs of a brain before orgasm and a brain during orgasm, it's like comparing a Christmas tree with just a few scattered light bulbs and one festooned with many strings of lights. With this imaging technology, researchers are starting to chart the effects of orgasm on the brain.

How does "sex-change" ("transsexual") surgery affect orgasms?

ACCORDING TO CHRISTINE MCGINN, who is one of the few surgeons in the United States who performs this type of surgery, some specific terminology is preferred. The surgery is referred to as "gender-confirming" surgery or "genital reassignment." *Transmen* refers to persons who undergo female-to-male surgery, and *transwomen* to persons who undergo male-to-female surgery.

For transwomen, the standard surgery is "penile inversion vaginoplasty." The surgery re-forms the main components of the penis into female proportions. The penile glans (the cone-shaped tip) is surgically reduced in size and sutured into position as a sensitive clitoris. Although many of its nerve endings are removed during this step, orgasmic ability remains intact. The testicles and erectile tissue of the penis are removed. The penile skin is left with an intact blood and nerve supply and is used to create the labia, clitoral hood, and vaginal wall. The vagina is created by surgically opening a space between the scrotum and the rectum and placing the inverted penile skin-tube within this space. The penile skin-tube is further lengthened by using a skin graft from the scrotum. The newly formed vagina ends blindly without a cervix and is located between the prostate and rectum. The prostate in transwomen remains in place after surgery and is an important source for orgasm, much like the G spot. Transwomen frequently report a decrease in desire as well as a change in character of their orgasms with estrogenic hormone therapy.

For transmen, there are two types of genital surgery: phalloplasty and metoidioplasty. Due to exclusion policies of many U.S. health insurance companies, the costly phalloplasty is not routinely performed in the United States; consequently, transmen undergo this surgery in other countries. While there are many techniques for phalloplasty, the basic method creates a penis from a flap of tissue from another area of the body (commonly, the forearm), using microsurgery. A nerve within the flap is attached to the ilioinguinal nerve and the clitoral branch of the pudendal nerve, allowing for sensation in the new phallus. The clitoris is incorporated into the base of the new phallus flap. The scrotum is created from the labia majora, and prosthetic silicon testicles are inserted.

In metoidioplasty, the clitoris is first enlarged by preparatory testosterone use. In the surgery, it is released from its attached ligaments in order to add length. Next, the urethra is extended and incorporated into the phallus. The dorsal nerves of the clitoris are left intact, and the individual is able to urinate from the standing position.

Transmen frequently report an increased desire as well as a change in character of their orgasms with androgenic hormone therapy. This may be related to the effects of hormone therapy on the frequency and quality of erectile tissue stimulation, but more research needs to be conducted in this area.

Anyone contemplating gender-confirming surgery should carefully consult with the surgeon about the expected changes and possible side effects. Psychological counseling is advisable to address the complexities of personal and social interactions.

How do machines and devices stimulate orgasms?

VARIOUS MACHINES AND DEVICES can be used as sex toys for recreational pleasure or as treatments to help overcome a sexual disorder. The simplest sex toys are vibrators, powered by battery or wall current. They are available in different sizes, shapes, textures, and colors, and are used by women and, although less so, by men.

Some vibrators are worn on the back of the hand, behind the fingers, so that genital contact is made by the vibrating fingers rather than by the vibrator itself. Other vibrators are applied directly to the genital region. This type of device varies in diameter of the stimulating head. Some women prefer to start out using a wider, rather than a narrower, vibrator for ease of stimulating the clitoris, and then, with practice, they make a transition to a narrower vibrator. The wider vibrators are also easier for a woman's partner to use. Vibrators that focus on clitoral stimulation are particularly appropriate for beginners or for individuals who want to avoid possible tearing of their hymen while enjoying self-stimulation. The hymen is a membrane inside the vagina near the vaginal entrance. The hymen only partially blocks the vaginal canal, thereby allowing the passage of menstrual flow.

Dildos resemble an erect penis in shape, size, and/or texture, and they may or may not contain a vibrator mechanism. They are made from a variety of materials, including pliable silicone or hard plastic, glass, or metal. They can stimulate the vaginal walls and give a woman a sense of penetration. The "Rabbit" is a Y-shaped dildo that is designed to stimulate the vagina internally at the same time as stimulating the clitoris externally. Another type of dildo is the "G spot stimulator," which is typically curved to apply pressure to the G spot, the anterior (belly-side) wall of the vagina, just behind the pubic bone. There are vibrating and nonvibrating designs. Some dildos have remote controls, which could be helpful for persons with physical limitations such as rheumatoid arthritis or obesity.

"Butt plugs" are small dildos designed specifically to stimulate the anus and rectum of women or men. They typically have a widened base at the end to prevent the dildo from inadvertently entering too deep into the rectum. Some butt plugs, such as Aneros, are devised to stimulate the prostate gland, which some men describe as pleasurable. Another type of sex toy for men is the artificial vagina. One example of this is the Fleshlight, which resembles a flashlight and contains a soft silicone vagina-shaped canal and an external vulva.

There are also devices that stimulate both partners simultaneously, such as penile ring vibrators, which the man puts around his penis to help him prolong his erection, and vibration from the ring stimulates his partner's clitoris during vaginal intercourse.

Some massagers, designed for use on the back, neck, or face, can also be used for sexual pleasure.

Other devices, such as Eros and vacuum constriction devices (the "sex pump," or VCD), increase blood flow to the genital area. The Eros is battery-powered, and the VCD has both mechanical and battery-powered models. The VCD was initially recommended for men who were experiencing erectile dysfunction as a complication of diabetes, prostate surgery, or spinal cord injury. The Eros, which is newer, was originally designed to help women who have arousal or orgasmic disorders related to low genital blood flow. Reports indicate that it's also useful for treating urinary urgency-frequency and urge incontinence ("overactive bladder") in women. While both Eros and the VCD are reported to be generally safe, you are advised to seek medical advice before embarking on use of these devices.

The Sybian is a large, electric motor-driven device that a woman sits astride. This device was made famous by its use on shows hosted by television and radio personality Howard Stern. The motor drives a thrusting dildo that can be moved at variable speed. The Venus is a large, electric motor-driven device that contains an artificial vagina into which a man inserts his penis; air is pushed and pulled rhythmically through the "vagina" at variable speed.

People use sex toys, including vibrators, for many different reasons. Some people might find it difficult or unacceptable to self-stimulate by hand, but don't feel the same way about self-stimulating with a device. In a sexual relationship, some may find it easier to give their partner pleasure using a device, rather than their hands. This may be especially true in elderly couples or in persons with physical limitations. Other people may just want to experiment with a new wrinkle in their sex life. It goes without saying that these devices won't solve relationship issues that may underlie interpersonal sexual difficulties. Casual sharing of sex toys should be viewed as being potentially as risky as unprotected sex, so they should not be shared. Sex toys should be cleaned according to the manufacturer's instructions.

In the United States and elsewhere, there are museums dedicated to these sexual devices. The Prague SexMachines Museum has more than two hundred objects and mechanical appliances available for view on its website, including machines from hundreds of years ago and devices with multiple functions, such as stimulating the clitoris while scratching the back. Another museum, the Museum of Sex, in New York City, exhibits a variety of patented sexual devices.

How can scientists tell whether animals have orgasms?

MALES OF EVERY SPECIES of mammal ejaculate, and many researchers have concluded that the activity seems to be rewarding, just as it is in humans. The orgasmic experience, however, must differ considerably among mammalian species, considering the great variability in ejaculatory patterns in terms of the amount of genital interaction required to ejaculate and the duration of the ejaculatory process itself. For a few species, we have precise information on the duration of the distinct behavioral events involved in mating (copulation, or coitus), including ejaculation.

In male rats, copulation lasts for an average of about one-third of a second, and then, after several of these brief copulations over the next few minutes, ejaculation occurs, lasting about two-thirds of a second. In rabbits, ejaculation occurs immediately following penile insertion; the contraction of the seminal vesicles, which produces the ejaculation, lasts about one second. If the perceptual experience of orgasm is directly related to these peripheral events, such as occurs in men, orgasm would last about one second. So, orgasm in rats and rabbits would be considerably shorter than in humans. The conscious perception of orgasm in most men has been timed to last twenty seconds or less.

One might wonder about the duration of the perceptual orgasm in a male pig, whose seminal emission and ejaculation lasts about five minutes! But what about the female pig? She stands still during these five minutes. Studies have shown that the male pig's breath immobilizes the female pig, and the essence in his breath has been identified as the biochemical 16-androstene. If this chemical is sprayed onto a female pig's nose, she stops moving. It is not known, however, whether the female pig stands immobilized for the five-minute duration of the male's ejaculation because of the effect of his breath or because it's rewarding to her, or perhaps both. (One might not be surprised if the breath of a copulating male pig had an immobilizing—or knockout—effect on a human, as well.)

The female pig exemplifies the problem of determining whether nonhuman females experience orgasm—we simply lack a good marker (such as ejaculation). The issue has been much debated, particularly among investigators interested in the idea that female orgasm is a specialized adaptation in humans, supposedly related to the reinforcement of bonding between the sexes. This position draws a clear distinction between women and other female primates. However, many data support the existence of female orgasm in other primates. Physiological responses identical to those occurring in women during orgasm have been observed in female monkeys of several species. In his book *Primate Sexuality*, Alan Dixson lists eight species of primates in which behavioral and physiological responses in females strongly suggest the presence of orgasm. Among the behavioral responses are a quick backward glance at the male, changes in facial expression ("climax face, open mouth, and grimaces"), and vocalizations. Among the physiological responses are uterine contractions, contractions of other tissues surrounding the vagina, and increased heart and respiratory rate.

Some researchers have claimed that other, nonprimate female mammals also experience orgasms, based on four kinds of evidence: (1) changes in heart rate, blood pressure, and respiration similar to those observed during orgasm in women, which have been recorded in several nonprimate mammalian species during copulation; (2) vaginal and uterine contractions in several species during copulation, comparable to those observed in women; (3) hormonal changes, some of them specifically associated with orgasm in women (such as release of prolactin), in nonprimate females; and (4) females' vocalizations during coitus.

Five

Orgasms and Health

Are orgasms good for our health?

THERE ARE CURRENTLY MORE than a million websites that discuss orgasms and health, so we know there's certainly a lot of interest in this topic. Overall, orgasms are evidently good for our health, even though they are not particularly effective at burning calories. An orgasm itself burns only two to three calories. However, a person can burn another fifty or more calories during the physical activity that leads to orgasm. One way to relate sexual activity to various forms of exercise is to compare "metabolic equivalents" (METs). One MET is defined as the amount of energy required to just sit quietly, which is about one calorie per kilogram (1 kilogram = 2.2 pounds) of body weight per hour. At this rate, a person who weighs 160 pounds would burn about 70 calories in one hour while sitting quietly or sleeping, which would be about 1,700 calories in twenty-four hours. Having sex with your partner uses about 5 METs. Having sex with someone who isn't your usual partner uses about 9 METs. Playing basketball also uses about 9 METs. Playing tennis uses 6 METs. Skiing uses 8 METs. Walking one mile uses 2.3 METs, and walking three miles uses 4.3 METs.

Research studies reviewed in a paper prepared by the Planned Parenthood Federation of America found that masturbation and partnered sexual activity may benefit many aspects of health and well-being, including longevity, immunity, reproductive health, and pain management. Some researchers have suggested that sexual activity may be correlated with a reduced risk of two of the leading causes of death in the western world: heart disease and cancer.

One study claimed that a steady and active sex life diminishes the negative physiological effects of aging and the risk for some diseases. Another study, which included 918 men between forty-five and fifty-nine years of age, probed the question in depth. The men were given a physical examination, including taking a medical history, measuring blood pressure, electrocardiogram, and cholesterol tests, and were asked about their frequency of orgasm. At a ten-year follow-up, it was found that the men who had reported having eight or more orgasms per month were twice as likely to be alive as the men who had less than one orgasm per month. The researchers concluded that "sexual activity seems to have a protective effect on men's health."

In the same group of 918 men, the researchers found that those who reported a high frequency of sexual intercourse were only half as likely to die of a heart attack (myocardial infarction, or MI—a blockage of blood flow to the heart muscle) as men who reported a low or intermediate frequency of orgasm.

There are not as many studies of women, but a study published in 1976 compared the sexual lives of 100 women hospitalized for heart attack (MI) with those of a group of 100 women of comparable age who were hospitalized for other reasons. Some of the questions about sexual life included the occurrence of "frigidity" (a 1970s term that is now considered obsolete). "Frigidity" was defined as a long-term lack of enjoyment of sexual intercourse, or a current inability to experience orgasm during intercourse, which created emotional dissatisfaction, or a current absence of orgasm, sexual enjoyment, and/or sexual intercourse due to a partner's illness or erectile dysfunction, which also created emotional dissatisfaction. The study found that the women with MI were more likely to be sexually "frigid" and sexually dissatisfied than the women hospitalized for other types of illness.

There is some evidence that male orgasms may protect women! Actually, the evidence is that pregnancy may afford a long-term protective effect against breast cancer. One researcher proposed in 1994 that a woman's immune response that protects against breast cancer may be triggered by antigenic proteins in her partner's sperm. The possible sperm effect was supported by a later study that found a woman's risk of breast cancer was associated with the number of lifetime male sexual partners she had: the more sex partners, the lower her risk of breast cancer. Although much less common, men also can have breast cancer. One study found that men with breast cancer have a lower frequency of orgasm than a comparison group of healthy men.

For men, two studies have provided evidence that the higher the frequency of ejaculations over many years, the lower the incidence of prostate cancer. In an Australian interview study of more than 2,000 men under the age of seventy, those who recalled having an average of four or more ejaculations per week during their twenties, thirties, and forties had a significantly lower (by one-third) risk of developing prostate cancer than men who reported an average of fewer than three ejaculations per week during the same age period. There was no association of prostate cancer with the number of sexual partners, suggesting that infectious factors did not account for the difference (it's well established that the greater the number of sexual partners, the higher the likelihood of acquiring a sexually transmitted infection, or STI).

In a questionnaire study of more than 50,000 American men ages forty to seventy-five, researchers found that the group of men who experienced many orgasms (at least twenty-one per month) were much less likely to have prostate cancer than the group who experienced moderate to low numbers of orgasms (seven or fewer per month). The researchers speculated that ejaculations may clear the prostate of potential carcinogenic substances and that psychological stress reduction resulting from ejaculation could reduce the release of "stress-related substances" (which could be related to eventual development of cancer) from the nerves that supply the prostate.

Orgasms may also serve as a sleep aid. It's well known that many men feel sleepy after experiencing an orgasm, and this seems to be less so in women, but one study found that many women use orgasm to induce sleep. The study reported that 32 percent of women who reported masturbating in the previous three months did so to facilitate falling asleep.

People experiencing pain may find that orgasms can offer some relief. In the 1970s researchers discovered that vaginal and cervical stimulation in laboratory animals blocks behavioral and brain responses to pain, a finding that led to similar studies with humans. The human studies showed that vaginal self-stimulation produces an increase in pain thresholds (ranging from 40 percent to more than 100 percent; an increase in pain threshold of 100 percent means that the woman has become half as sensitive to the pain). However, these women do not "go numb." Their sense of touch is not diminished, just their reaction to pain. A later study found that pleasurable stimulation of all areas of the genitals elevates pain thresholds. The most effective area for increasing pain threshold when stimulated is the area of the G spot. Orgasm produces the greatest increase in pain thresholds. This effect has not been measured in men, although anecdotal evidence that men become insensitive to pain at the time of orgasm has been described for many years.

Do orgasms reduce stress?

YES, THERE IS RESEARCH evidence that sexual activity and orgasm can reduce stress. A study of 2,632 American women found that 39 percent of those who masturbated reported doing so to relax. When a person experiences orgasm, the hormone oxytocin is released from nerve cells in the hypothalamus (a region of the brain) into the bloodstream. Low levels of oxytocin in the blood are correlated with a relatively high incidence of tension and anxiety disorders, whereas higher levels are correlated with reduced responsiveness to stress.

In addition to the physiological role of orgasm in reducing stress, orgasmic pleasure in a mutually loving relationship can benefit the mental health of the partners and the quality of the relationship. But we must note that if individuals attempt to stimulate orgasms specifically to achieve relaxation afterward, this may place the partners under performance pressure—which could intensify stress rather than reduce it.

In rare cases, individuals have been forced to have orgasms by a sexual abuser or during a sexual assault. Following such abuse or assault, it's possible that orgasmic sensations intensify the individual's stress rather than providing a sense of relief. People who experience increased stress when having an orgasm should see a sexuality counselor or psychosexual therapist (ideally, one who is experienced in dealing with victims of sexual abuse).

Can an orgasm cause a heart attack?

When a former vice president of the United States, Nelson A. Rockefeller, died of a heart attack during a sexual encounter in a hotel with a much younger woman, it triggered great interest among the public. People wanted to know whether "death in the saddle" was common or rare. The answer is that it is rare. In one study of 5,559 cases of sudden death in men, fewer than 20 deaths occurred during a sexual act. In general, it seems that the exertion associated with sexual activity is more the culprit than is the actual orgasm.

According to one medical examiner, "death in the saddle" follows a pattern in which "the deceased [man] is usually married; he is with a non-spouse in unfamiliar surroundings after a big meal with alcohol." (Unfortunately, so far, most scientific articles on the incidence of "death by sex" focus on men.) One study reported that 70 percent of twenty coital (sexual intercourse) deaths recorded had occurred during extra-marital intercourse. This suggests that added stresses could have been involved in these deaths. The researchers cited another study in which coroners estimated that "acute coronary insufficiency resulting from coitus is a fact, but the incidence rate is no more than three out of every 500 subjects with heart disease." The researchers concluded that "it is obvious that coital death is a rare occurrence, and that reports of coital death of a middle aged, middle-class, male patient with heart disease who engages in sexual activity with his wife of 20 or more years in their own bedroom is even rarer."

In a more recent review, the same researchers caution that the increases in heart rate and blood pressure that occur during intercourse might "precipitate the fracture or erosion of a vulnerable atherosclerotic plaque with subsequent thrombus (clot) formation and arterial occlusion." However, they cite a survey of more than 1,700 patients in which "sexual activity was noted to be a potential triggering event prior to MI in only 1.5 percent of patients." These authors concluded that "absolute risk caused by sexual activity is considerably low: one chance in one million healthy individuals. Cardiac rehabilitation and exercise training programs can reduce incidence of chest pain (angina pectoris) during sexual activity." One medical heart expert recently recommended a gradual increase in sexual exertion after a heart attack. The recommendation is to resume sexual activity slowly, over a period of six or more weeks, starting with gentle caressing, then mutual genital manipulation, and eventually intercourse, as long as no medical symptoms, such as chest pain, occur as exertion increases.

Can orgasms cause headaches?

YES. SOME MEN AND women suffer from "pre-orgasmic headache," which is characterized by a dull ache in the head and neck associated with muscle contraction in the jaw muscles that increases with sexual excitement. An "orgasmic headache" has also been described—a sudden severe ("explosive" or "thunderclap") headache that occurs at orgasm produced by masturbation or intercourse. Some, but not all, men and women who have orgasmic headaches also suffer from migraines. The orgasmic headache is said to last for minutes, hours, or even days. To be on the safe side, when experiencing such severe headaches, the individual should see a doctor to rule out the possibility of an aneurysm (ballooned, locally weakened blood vessel) or a burst blood vessel supplying the meninges (the membranes that form a capsule around the brain and spinal cord).

Another type of headache associated with orgasm has been described as "ice-pick-like," with the pain felt in the face. Someone who experiences this type of headache should be tested for possible epileptic activity or compression of, or stretching of, the spinal cord, which may be related to prior trauma, a tumor, or a congenital condition. Another possible cause of this type of orgasmic headache is constriction of blood vessels that convey blood to the meninges.

Some physicians suggest that orgasmic headaches are similar to headaches after exercise, which are related to a temporary rise in blood pressure, muscle spasm of the neck or scalp, or dilation of blood vessels in the meninges. Orgasmic headache also has similarities to headache after the procedure known as a "spinal tap," which may be due to reduced pressure of the spinal fluid after the sample of fluid is removed.

Relief from orgasmic headache has been obtained with a class of drugs known as triptans. Triptans (which are also effective against migraine headaches) are reported to reduce the duration and severity of orgasmic headaches and even to prevent orgasmic headaches when they are taken thirty minutes before intercourse. Propanolol (a type of drug known as a beta-blocker) and calcium-channel blockers are other headache medicines that can be effective in preventing orgasmic headaches.

What causes "blue balls"?

THERE IS SURPRISINGLY LITTLE research on this widely discussed issue. The scientific literature through the 1990s is a barren shelf, but a medical discussion of "blue balls" was started with publication of a case report in the major medical journal *Pediatrics* in 2000. The authors (two physicians) wrote that "'blue balls' is a widely used colloquialism describing testicular and scrotal pain after high, sustained sexual arousal unrelieved because of lack of orgasm and ejaculation. It is remarkable that the medical literature completely lacks acknowledgment of this condition." The authors described a case of a fourteen-year-old who came to the emergency room with testicular-scrotal pain that had persisted for more than an hour. The boy reported experiencing the pain previously, when he was petting with his girlfriend; on neither occasion did he ejaculate and on both occasions the pain started immediately after stopping foreplay. An examination found that the boy had no current or prior relevant pathology, and the pain subsided after an hour in the emergency room. On subsequent telephone follow-up, he revealed that he'd started having sexual intercourse with his girlfriend, with no further episodes of testicular-scrotal pain.

The authors of this report suggested that the pain in cases of this sort might result from the lack of orgasmic resolution, which could lead to insufficient draining of blood from the genitals and/or increased pressure in the epididymal tubes, through which sperm and fluid are normally transported away from the testicles. "The treatment is sexual release," the authors wrote, "or perhaps straining to move a very heavy object" (a straining procedure known as the "Valsalva maneuver").

This report stimulated a letter to the editor of the journal, which read: "we wonder whether the authors' suggestion that 'straining to move a very heavy object' is the first choice . . . As this condition is coming to light in a highly respected pediatric journal, perhaps we should resurrect the advice of former Surgeon General Jocelyn Elders and teach masturbation in the schools. This novel idea, which led to her removal from office, should have been implemented yesterday." Jocelyn Elders,

M.D., was appointed U.S. surgeon general by President Bill Clinton and served for fifteen months in his administration, until she was forced to resign in 1994 as a direct result of suggesting that schools should consider teaching masturbation to students as a means of preventing sexually transmitted diseases.

In response to the letter's suggestion that sexual release is an effective treatment for blue balls, another letter appeared: "What are the ethical implications of such a statement? Will young men demand sexual satisfaction of their partners as essential medical therapy? Do the authors condone self-treatment? What about potential adverse effects of treatment, such as blindness and palmar hypertrichosis [hairiness] (personal communications, our mothers)? What are the ethical and/or medical responsibilities for the health care team in treating young men in an urgent care setting? And if treatment is rendered, are there appropriate diagnostic and treatment codes for billing purposes?"

The authors of the original article responded in yet another letter to the editor of *Pediatrics*: "A 70-year-old retired college professor told us . . . [that] in the 1940s a practicing physician taught him and his fellow eighth-graders about sexuality, including 'lover's nuts.' The doctor told them that masturbation was at times a legitimate medical treatment." They continued: "In no way should the pain of blue balls be an excuse to inappropriately advance a sexual relationship. As part of sexual education, we might teach that sexual urges are natural, abstinence is a real choice, and sexual decisions ought never to be based on coercion or exploitation." They concluded with the droll pun: "blue balls is real, and a cure is coming."

In a subsequent commentary on the dialogue, an engineer, L. N. Ludovici (in a letter with coauthor J. Arndt) wrote: "I have had a vasectomy and noticed that I no longer get blue balls with prolonged sexual excitement if there is no release by ejaculation. Instead, I feel pain along the path of the vas deferens down to the point where it is sealed off. Indeed, with palpation of the vas deferens, it feels swollen. If blue balls were caused by blood engorgement in the testicles I would still get it since the vasectomy did not cut the blood vessels. I conclude that blue balls is caused not by blood engorgement, but by seminal fluid engorgement. I theorize that since the fraction of the seminal fluid that is produced outside of the testicles has nowhere to go, it backs down the vas deferens into the normally connected testes and swells the whole system to the point of pain."

Until someone undertakes a more serious analysis of blue balls syndrome, it will most likely remain a controversial, and much discussed, phenomenon.

What is the effect of cancer and its treatment on orgasm?

MOST OFTEN, ORGASM REMAINS intact for men and women who have been diagnosed with or have been treated for and survived cancer. However, it is a common complaint of cancer survivors that they find it difficult to restart their sexual life after they have been treated for their cancer. After treatment, orgasm may become delayed or more difficult to experience for reasons related to medications or the emotional adjustment to cancer, or both. The medications and emotional adjustment can also lead to a common sexual problem for people with cancer: loss of desire for sexual activity. The loss of desire seems to affect men and women equally. In general, cancer patients undergoing treatment and recent cancer survivors commonly find rigorous physical activities fatiguing, which may also reduce interest in engaging in sexual activity.

Other cancer-related sexual problems commonly experienced are erectile dysfunction in men and dyspareunia (pain during vaginal intercourse) in women. These problems could be due to treatments such as radiation therapy to the genital area or surgical procedures such as hysterectomy and bilateral salpingo-oophorectomy, in which the uterus, cervix, ovaries, and fallopian tubes are removed.

Surgical procedures related to cancer may affect the nerve and blood supply to the genital region, interfering with stimulation of arousal and erection in men, lubrication and vaginal and cervical sensation in women, and orgasm in both men and women. In the case of dyspareunia, a course of dilation therapy (in which the woman uses a graded series of dilators, from finger size to penis size, for daily massage of the vaginal opening and walls to ease penile penetration), use of lubricants, and use of sedatives may help the woman become more comfortable with vaginal intercourse.

As a result of total hysterectomy (removal of the uterus and cervix), women may experience changes in genital sensations due to pain or to loss of sensation and numbness, as well as a decreased ability to experience orgasm. Premature ovarian failure as a result of chemotherapy or pelvic radiation therapy is also often a preliminary to sexual disorders, particularly when hormone replacement is inadvisable ("contraindicated") because the growth of the cancerous cells is hormonally sensitive. Premature ovarian failure resulting from chemotherapy or radiation precipitates the onset of menopausal symptoms due to the sudden loss of estrogen and androgen normally produced by the ovaries. These symptoms include vaginal atrophy (shrinkage), thinning of the vulvar tissues and vagina, loss of tissue elasticity, decreased vaginal lubrication, hot flashes, increased frequency of urinary tract infections, mood swings, fatigue, and irritability. When not contraindicated because of cancer risk, physician-prescribed replacement of the ovarian hormones—by hormone patch, pill, or injection—can diminish and control these symptoms.

Men who undergo treatment for prostate cancer (chemical, surgical, and/or radiation) may experience ejaculation that is delayed, inhibited, or "retrograde" (the ejaculated fluid goes into the bladder rather than out through the urethra, due to failure of the urethra's internal sphincter). In some cases, ejaculation may not occur at all. Among men with prostate cancer who have received anti-androgen therapy ("chemical castration," which is done to decrease the normal prostate-stimulatory effect of androgens), about 80 percent report a profound decrease in sexual interest, typically accompanied by erectile dysfunction and difficulty experiencing orgasms.

Relationship problems, such as a change of "power" between partners, may also occur following a cancer diagnosis and treatment. With the new role for one partner as caretaker of the partner with cancer, the personal interactions may change dramatically, creating tension and conflict in the couple's emotional and sexual relationship. In a common misconception, the partner of the cancer patient erroneously believes that if he or she overstimulates or puts too much pressure on the partner with cancer, this will cause a relapse (return) of the disease. So he or she withholds such stimulation or does not make sexual requests. Such overly cautious behavior might lead to weakening of the couple's emotional and sexual relationship.

Depending on the type of cancer and its severity, surgeons have developed nerve-sparing procedures that allow them to remove cancerous tumors and other structures while minimizing damage to sexual function. For example, for men with colorectal cancer (cancer of the colon and rectum), development of surgical techniques that spare the hypogastric and pelvic plexus nerves has allowed patients to largely retain erectile and ejaculatory function and orgasm. Similar nerve-sparing surgical procedures can also be used in the case of prostate cancer, depending on its location and severity. We are surprised that the medical literature seems to offer only a few reports of nerve-sparing surgery for women who undergo hysterectomy.

Does hysterectomy affect orgasms?

A HYSTERECTOMY (THE REMOVAL OF the uterus and, in a total hysterectomy, the cervix and the uterus) may affect a woman's ability to experience orgasm in three main ways. First, hysterectomy eliminates or reduces pain and excessive menstrual bleeding. If the pain and bleeding were negatively affecting a woman's enjoyment of sex, then the hysterectomy could improve her sexual experience. Second, the surgery can affect the sensations from the sexual organs directly by damaging blood and nerve supplies, or the medication that follows the surgery can interfere with the neurotransmitters in the brain that control sexual feeling and the ability to have an orgasm. So, there is the potential for a decline in sexual sensations and desire. Third, any surgery can have a profound psychological impact.

The nerves that convey sensation from the clitoris are likely to remain undamaged by hysterectomy, so clitoral sensation is unlikely to be affected. However, the nerves that convey sensation from the vagina are more likely to be damaged by the surgery, and this could reduce the woman's ability to experience orgasm. In the case of a total hysterectomy, in which the cervix is also removed, cervical sensation is eliminated, and for some women, both vaginal and cervical stimulation are an important component of their orgasmic experience.

The many studies that are available on the effects of hysterectomy on a woman's sexual experience don't paint a clear picture of the outcomes, mainly because they fail to report on women's preferred regions of genital stimulation, and the different regions can be differently affected by the surgery.

Besides hysterectomy, do other female genital surgeries affect orgasms?

HYSTERECTOMY MAY BE THE most commonly discussed surgery affecting female genitals, but there are many other surgeries that may affect a woman's ability to experience orgasm. These other "pelvic surgeries" include, but are not limited to, oophorectomy (removal of the ovaries), cystectomy (partial or complete removal of the urinary bladder), vulvectomy (which might involve the removal of the top layer of the vulval skin affected by cancer or, in severe cases, the entire vulva and deep tissues, including the clitoris), and abdomino-perineal resection (a radical surgical procedure in which the anus, rectum, and sigmoid colon are removed to treat cancer located very low in the rectum or in the anus, close to the sphincter—the muscle that keeps closed and opens the anus). If the surgeon is successful in retaining adequate blood supply and preserving healthy nerves, the effects of these surgeries on sexual activity and orgasm may be minimal. Conversely, disturbance in the function of the blood or nerve supply could lead to a sexual disorder. If you are to undergo surgical treatment of this sort, it's important to inform your surgeon beforehand about the importance to you of retaining your sexual function. The surgeon will then take extra care when working on these nerves, veins, and arteries.

Does prostate surgery affect orgasms?

IN SOME CASES, YES. Removal of the prostate gland (prostatectomy) is one of the most common male pelvic surgeries. This surgery can damage nerves and blood vessels and, at a minimum, removes an important male sex organ. The risks associated with prostate surgery include occasional or total loss of erection, loss of ability to ejaculate, expulsion of urine at orgasm ("orgasm-associated incontinence"), painful ejaculation, and sexual desire disorder (decrease or loss of sexual desire). Men may be at least as affected psychologically by prostate surgery as women are by hysterectomy, because the effects of prostate surgery can be more externally evident—possibly affecting erection, penetration, and ejaculation.

Men with an intact prostate who experience pain at the point of ejaculation or immediately afterward may have prostatitis (an inflammation of the prostate gland that develops gradually), benign prostatic hyperplasia (enlargement of the prostate gland, which occurs with age), or ejaculatory duct obstruction. These are medical conditions that may be treatable with medication, but they may require surgery.

Men facing prostate surgery should be frank with their doctors, asking questions about the potential consequences involved in the surgery. Recent improvements in surgical techniques have greatly reduced the risks to men's sexual functioning.

Besides prostate surgery, do other male genital surgeries affect orgasms?

THERE ARE MANY OTHER forms of surgery in men that can profoundly affect orgasm. These include abdomino-perineal resection (in which the anus, rectum, and sigmoid colon are removed), cystectomy (partial or total removal of the urinary bladder), vesiculectomy (partial or total removal of the seminal vesicles), urethrectomy (removal of the urethra), orchidectomy (removal of one or both testicles), and penectomy (partial or total removal of the penis).

Are there surgeries that can improve a man's chance of experiencing orgasm?

FAILURE TO DEVELOP AN erection obviously can mechanically prevent a man from experiencing orgasms from vaginal intercourse. If, despite lack of erection, the man has penile sensation, surgical implants can make the penis sufficiently rigid for orgasms to be stimulated through intercourse.

There are two major types of surgical implant. One type is a semi-rigid, malleable rod (like a goose-neck lamp) that makes the penis rigid (two rods are implanted). The penis can be raised or lowered by bending the rods, although the circumference of the penis does not change. The other type consists of two inflatable cylinders that are implanted in the penis. A reservoir of liquid is implanted in the abdomen or scrotum, and a pump is implanted in the scrotum. When the pump is squeezed, the liquid from the reservoir fills the two cylinders and the penis becomes erect. Squeezing a release bar near the pump returns the fluid to the reservoir when an erection is no longer desired. The advantages of the surgical implants are a long-lasting effect and a high degree of satisfaction among men who have them. The disadvantages include irreversibility, invasiveness, and the potential for surgical complications and mechanical failure.

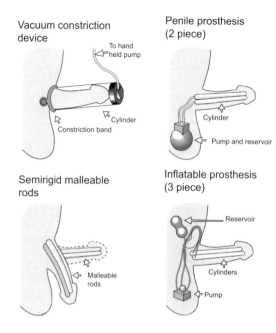

Prosthetic devices for producing penile erection. The two main types of surgically implanted devices designed to enable penetrative intercourse are the malleable rods (lower left) and the hydraulic pump plus inflatable rods (upper and lower right). The malleable rods can be bent into an erect position when desired, supporting the penis. In the pump-and-reservoir devices, inflatable rods are implanted in the penis, the pump is placed in the scrotum, and the hydraulic reservoir is implanted into the scrotum or nearby. The pump is activated manually, inflating the cylinders in the penis to produce an erection. The nonsurgical suction device, with constriction band (upper left), is shown for comparison. (Adapted from image courtesy Dr. Gorm Wagner)

Another type of surgery in men with erectile dysfunction involves the blood vessels. According to Thomas Lue, young men who have inadequate penile blood flow can be treated surgically to increase arterial inflow and decrease venous outflow, enabling them to experience erections and orgasms from vaginal intercourse.

How do brain injuries or spinal cord injuries affect orgasms?

THERE ARE REPORTS OF "hypersexuality" produced by some types of brain damage. The basis for the hypersexuality may be a combination of loss of discrimination of appropriate sexual objects, loss of social inhibitions, and increased sexual desire.

There was a report in 1955 of a nineteen-year-old man with temporal lobe epilepsy that was resistant to medication. He underwent surgical removal of parts of his brain (anterior portion of the temporal lobes, anterior portion of the hippocampus, and the amygdala, on both sides of his brain). After the surgery, "He picked up objects . . . the same object again and again . . . [and] displayed to the doctor, with satisfaction, that he had spontaneous erections followed by masturbation and orgasm . . . became exhibitionistic . . . wanted to show his sexual organ erect to all doctors . . . [and] showed indifference [to women] in contrast with his behavior before the operation . . . Homosexual tendencies . . . were soon noticed . . . [and he practiced] self-abuse several times a day."

Two surgeons in the 1940s noted increased sexuality in about 25 percent of their patients who had undergone frontal lobotomy, a procedure mainly used to treat depression or psychosis before the advent of effective medications. The controversial physicians Walter Freeman and James Watts, who performed more than 500 frontal lobotomies in the 1940s, commented that "it would seem that the postoperative inertia manifested by some patients reduces the tendency of the individual to seek sexual gratification. On the other hand, the suppression of the restraining forces may lead to a freer expression of the personality along sexual lines." In the latter case, in which an effect of the surgery was to relax social inhibitions, patients were described as making inappropriate advances to members of their own and the other sex and masturbating in public. With the introduction of antidepressant and antipsychotic drugs after the 1950s, frontal lobotomy became obsolete.

There are several reports of hypersexuality after surgery that encroached on the septal region of the patient's brain. The behavior patterns were similar to those occurring after frontal lobotomy: socially inappropriate sexual advances to others, masturbation in public, demands for sexual intercourse many times a day—all behavior patterns that were not present before the surgery.

Different parts of the brain excite and inhibit sexual activity in humans, normally maintaining a balance between the two tendencies. However, when specific regions of the brain are damaged by trauma or surgery, an imbalance can occur that results in an increase or decrease in sexual motivation and behavior. Specifying the brain regions affected by the trauma or surgery is not precise enough to conclude exactly which brain regions control which sexuality functions or to predict the ways in which sexuality might be affected by an individual case of brain trauma or surgery.

Women and men with spinal cord injury suffer problems of bowel and bladder control, spasticity (uncontrollable, powerful contractions of leg and back muscles), and, depending on the level of the injury, the possibility of sudden elevation of blood pressure with associated severe headache. The reduced genital sensation that results from the damage to the sensory pathways from the genitals to the brain adds to the distress. Sexual desire, however, is often unaffected in people with spinal cord injury.

We give here just a short and necessarily oversimplified account—oversimplified because there are many individual differences, depending on physical, physiological, emotional, and interpersonal factors.

In men, complete spinal cord injury blocks signals passing from the brain down the spinal cord to the genitals (*complete* means that there is no voluntary motor control or sensory awareness below the injury site). For these men, sexual arousal such as by "psychogenic" factors—erotic visual, verbal, thought, fantasy—or any stimulation originating in the brain rather than in the genitals cannot be transmitted to the genitals. If the complete spinal cord injury is near the base of the spinal cord, which is just below the last rib, erection, ejaculation, and orgasm in response to physical stimulation of the penis may also be blocked, due to damage to the nerves that carry genital sensation to the spinal cord. However, if the damage is higher up in the spinal cord, erection in response to physical stimulation of the penis may be possible, even if ejaculation and orgasm are blocked. If the spinal cord damage is still higher, near the level of the upper ribs or above, then erection and ejaculation in response to physical penile stimulation may be possible, although orgasm may be blocked.

There are many exceptions to these generalizations. If the spinal cord injury is *incomplete*, sensory pathways from the genitals to the brain may be variably intact or damaged. Some reports describe men with spinal cord injury who experience orgasm from genital stimulation. It may be possible to induce ejaculation, if not by manual penile stimulation, then by vibrator or by electrical stimulation with a rectal probe. Viable sperm may be obtained by these methods, which can be used to impregnate the partner, at least by in vitro fertilization.

Even in cases of complete spinal cord injury in which genital sensory awareness is absent, caressing of other sensate body regions can elicit orgasms, such as stimulation of the hypersensitive skin region near the level of the spinal cord injury, in the "right" way by the "right" person. Other potentially erogenous body regions above the level of the injury include the nipples, ears, lips, tongue, face, and neck.

For women who have a severed spinal cord near the level of the nipples or above, research shows, surprisingly, that stimulation of the vagina and cervix (whose sensory nerves connect to the spinal cord below the site of injury) can induce orgasm. These women have no sensation of the clitoris, vulva, and labia, because of their injury. But the pair of vagus nerves convey enough sensory activity from the cervix and vagina directly to the brain (outside the spinal cord) to stimulate orgasms. The vagus nerves travel near the intestines, along the esophagus (the tube that connects the mouth to the stomach), up through the chest and neck, and into the brain. We don't know whether every woman with a complete spinal cord injury will have a functional vagus nerve pathway. But for a woman with spinal cord injury who desires sexual stimulation, it's worth exploring whether she still has sensory awareness to physical stimulation of the deep vagina and cervix.

What treatments are there for erectile dysfunction?

Erectile dysfunction (ED), previously called "impotence," has numerous causes and many treatment options. The dysfunction can be lifelong or situational. The cause may be organic, psychological, mixed, or unknown. "Complete erectile dysfunction" is defined as the total inability to obtain or maintain erections during sexual stimulation, as well as the absence of nocturnal (nighttime) erections. There are also lesser degrees of ED. To produce an erection, certain penile blood vessels dilate, allowing extra blood to be pumped into the penis, which causes the penis to expand. The outgoing blood vessels are squeezed partially shut as the penis becomes engorged with blood, causing less blood to flow out. The increased inflow combined with the decreased outflow of blood results in an erection. In ED, there is insufficient blood flow into the penis (and, sometimes, too much outflow). The lack of a "backup of blood" results in a penis that is either flaccid or insufficiently rigid.

Before the U.S. Food and Drug Administration (FDA) approved Viagra (sildenafil) in 1998, very few men with ED reported this problem to a physician or sex therapist. Today, Viagra, Levitra (vardenafil HCl), Cialis (tadalafil), and related medications are commonly prescribed, and many men feel comfortable telling their doctor they have a problem related to erection. Doctors have also become more comfortable asking their patients about their sex life, something that may have been viewed as inappropriate in years past.

It was long believed that about 80 percent of cases of ED were psychological in origin, and many, if not most, women believed it was their fault if their partner had ED, because the woman felt she was no longer attractive or sufficiently sexually arousing. However, we now know that a large majority of cases of ED are due to medical factors related to the man.

Erectile dysfunction can be associated with a wide range of medical conditions and psychological problems caused by depression, relationship difficulties, and even employment changes. Physiological bases for ED include vascular problems as a consequence of high blood pressure, diabetes and diabetes-related nerve damage, elevated levels of cholesterol and other lipids, multiple sclerosis, Parkinson disease, various surgical procedures, even prolonged bicycle riding, and side effects associated with prescription or nonprescription drug use. Smoking, alcohol, and stress can also contribute to ED.

In recommending a treatment, doctors must consider the needs and priorities of the man and his sex partner(s), which will be influenced by cultural, social, ethnic, religious, and national factors. Men with ED and their partner(s) should select the best treatment for their sexual concerns, after receiving appropriate education that includes information on sexuality and all treatment options. In evaluating the various treatments for ED, a family's traditions, ethnicity, and socioeconomic conditions, as well as the man's and his partner's preferences, expectations, and psychological status, must be carefully weighed. This is a couple's issue, not just one man's issue.

Depending on the underlying reasons for the ED, the following treatments are among the individual's and couple's options.

Psychological and sex therapy

There are four major components of sex therapy for ED: (1) anxiety reduction and desensitization; (2) cognitive-behavioral interventions; (3) increased sexual stimulation; and (4) interpersonal assertiveness and couple's communication training. Men with ED and their partners are often resistant to psychological interventions, because of the potential implication that the problem is "all in his head" or that the man is purposefully avoiding sexual intimacy.

For some cases of ED, a combined approach might work best. Men with ED or their partners frequently have other sexual or relationship concerns, psychological distress, or partner conflict, and these can best be addressed with a combination of medical and sex therapy interventions.

In some cases, cognitive-behavioral therapy could be useful. During this form of therapy some exercises are assigned to the person to help him gain confidence and a sense of control over his body. One of these exercises is to slowly stimulate the penis to an erection (by self-stimulation or by the partner). As soon as an erection is produced, the stimulation should be stopped. Then, after a few seconds, when the penis is semi-erect or flaccid, the stimulation should begin again and the same process repeated. On the third occasion, the stimulation could be continued with hand or oral stimulation to bring the person to orgasm and ejaculation. This is an effective psychological exercise that demonstrates to the man that he can produce an erection whenever, and as many times as, he desires, and he need not "use it or lose it." Performed in conjunction with a caring and loving relationship, this technique can be very effective. It is one of the techniques that are widely used in combination with other exercises to help men with psychosexual bases for their ED, such as performance anxiety.

Muscle exercise

Researchers in Europe found that if men with ED went on a special exercise program, this was just as successful in improving erection capacity as taking Viagra. This research group found that more than 80 percent of the men who exercised reported better erections, compared with 74 percent of those taking Viagra and 18 percent of the placebo group (the group taking a pill that looked like Viagra but contained only inactive ingredients; use of a placebo group is standard procedure in well-controlled clinical studies). The exercise program was aimed at improving blood supply around the pelvic region, buttocks, and upper leg muscles by means of squatting and leg lifts. In another study of men who followed an exercise program to strengthen their pelvic floor muscles, erections were highly improved. This success with exercise is especially true if the ED is due to mild leakage in the veins that drain the penis, in which case the penis does not sufficiently maintain a backup of blood to keep an erection.

Nontraditional treatments

Several over-the-counter products are available for treatment of ED, but most of them have not been tested in adequately controlled research studies and the results published in professional journals. One product that has been appropriately studied and positive results reported is ArginMax for Men. It contains gingko biloba, Korean ginseng, American ginseng, l-arginine, and vitamins. A 1994 study reported that this product improved men's ability to maintain an erection during intercourse and improved their satisfaction with their overall sex life, compared with men who received a placebo.

Medical treatments

Medical treatments for ED can be divided into three major categories:

1. Oral pharmacological agents
2. Local (nonsurgical and mechanical) therapies
3. Surgical treatments

Oral pharmacological agents. Several oral pharmacological agents are approved for this use, of which the most commonly used are the PDE-5 inhibitors (phosphodiesterase type-5 inhibitors, a name that refers to their mechanism of action). Viagra, Levitra, and Cialis are PDE-5 inhibitors. These drugs do not produce sexual desire; instead, they facilitate erection of the penis in response to cognitive (psychogenic) or physical sexual stimulation. Basically, these drugs open the blood vessels that supply the penis and thus allow more blood to enter. Men may experience side effects from these drugs, including headache, facial flushing, and visual problems. Furthermore, the blood vessel–dilating effect of these drugs can add to the blood vessel–dilating effect of nitroglycerine-type drugs—including illegal drugs such as "poppers" (amyl nitrate)—to produce a dangerous and sometimes fatal drop in blood pressure.

Other oral products are available, but the PDE-5 inhibitors are the most commonly used. Some other types of drugs are currently under clinical investigation.

Local (nonsurgical and mechanical) therapies. Injection of Alprostadil (a prostaglandin) through a fine needle directly into the corpora cavernosa (the spongy erectile tissues that form the body of the penis) is one treatment that brings about a rapid erection. The drug is self-injected, or injected by a partner. Alprostadil relaxes smooth muscles, dilating arterial blood vessels and so improving blood flow into the penis. The drug can also be applied in the form of a semi-solid pellet that is inserted, with a special applicator, directly into the urethra (the channel in the penis that conveys the ejaculate and urine). Some men report pain with this method, and there are rare cases of low blood pressure and dizziness. It's recommended that if the female partner is, or may be, pregnant, a condom should be used with this type of therapy. Some research suggests the pellet method is not as effective as the injection method.

Vacuum constriction devices (VCDs) are widely available, including over the counter (without a prescription) in some countries. They consist of a plastic cylinder with a pump attached. The man places the cylinder over his penis and pumps the air out, drawing blood into the penis and creating an erection. A plastic ring, which is supplied with the VCD, is then placed around the base of the penis to maintain the erection. Although VCDs are cumbersome to use, they are nonpharmacological and may appeal to some men who prefer to avoid taking medications.

Surgical treatments. Surgical implants in the penis are among several surgical procedures for the treatment of ED (see, earlier in this chapter, "Are there surgeries that can improve a man's chance of experiencing orgasm?"). Non-invasive treatments should be attempted first.

Does Viagra help women experience orgasm?

VIAGRA AND SIMILAR DRUGS (Cialis, Levitra) that are used to treat erectile dysfunction—the PDE-5 inhibitors—have also been tested for use in treating women with sexual disorders.

Although the effectiveness of Viagra on women's sexual desire and orgasmic response remains controversial, most studies show that this drug increases blood flow into the clitoris. The side effects, as in men, are relatively minor, but there are health risks associated with taking any drug, and PDE-5 inhibitors in particular. The manufacturer of Viagra discontinued testing it in women, and the FDA has not approved it for use in women. Certainly, no one—men or women—should take these drugs without careful consultation with their doctor about the risks and potential benefits.

Does vaginal dryness affect orgasms?

WHEN THE VAGINA IS inadequately lubricated, it can feel itchy and irritated. Vaginal dryness may make some activities uncomfortable, and it can make vaginal intercourse less pleasurable. It can cause pain or light bleeding with sexual intercourse, and it may cause urinary frequency or urgency because of the thinning of the lining of the urethra and the vagina. During menopause, vaginal dryness is a common cause of discomfort or pain for the woman, and perhaps for the man, during vaginal intercourse. Burning and pain during vaginal intercourse can begin long before a gynecologist is able to detect changes in vaginal tissue. Of course, vaginal dryness can greatly reduce a woman's pleasure and interfere with her ability to experience orgasm.

Vaginal dryness is a common condition that can affect women of all ages, although it occurs most often during and after menopause. It can also be caused as a side effect of drugs such as antihistamines and decongestants, which are taken to dry up the mucous membranes in the nose. In relation to menopause, reduced estrogen levels are the main cause of vaginal dryness. Estrogen, a hormone secreted mainly by the ovaries but also by the adrenals, helps keep the vaginal tissue healthy by promoting normal vaginal lubrication, and it helps keep the tissue elastic and normally acidic. These are natural defenses against vaginal and urinary tract infection. Estrogen levels decrease around the time of menopause, and the vaginal lining becomes thinner and more fragile. Reduced vaginal lubrication may also occur as a result of childbirth, breastfeeding, treatment for cancer, surgical removal of the ovaries, and smoking.

Douching, the process of cleaning the vagina with a liquid preparation, disrupts the normal chemical balance in the vagina and may cause inflammation. This can cause the vagina to feel dry and irritated. Most health care professionals recommend that women should not douche.

Medical diagnosis of vaginal dryness is made by a pelvic examination performed by a health care practitioner. A sample of cervical cells or vaginal secretions may be taken for microscopic examination. Low estrogen levels, which may be the basis for vaginal dryness, can most reliably be determined by a blood test for FSH (follicle-stimulating hormone). For women who are still menstruating, estrogen levels in the blood vary with the time of the menstrual cycle, and tests for estrogen are not as reliable as measurement of FSH levels in blood, which increase as estrogen levels decrease.

There are several self-care and medical treatments that can help reduce vaginal dryness. If the vaginal dryness is due to a lack of adequate estrogen and if the following self-care measures don't correct the problem, vaginal estrogen therapy may be ordered by prescription.

Self-care measures

The most commonly used water-based lubricants are Astroglide and K-Y jelly. They lubricate the vagina for several hours and are safe for use with latex products such as condoms and dental dams. Vaginal moisturizers such as Replens last longer than lubricants. They may decrease dryness for up to three days with a single application. Women should probably avoid many of the other products that claim to help, as very few have been properly tested and evaluated.

Oil-based products such as Vaseline or massage oil may produce vaginal dryness. They should not be used with latex condoms and other latex products because they can cause deterioration of the latex. It's advisable to avoid other products that have not been studied through standard scientific research procedures. The vagina may become irritated by application of vinegar, yogurt, hand lotions, soaps, and bubble baths, and by other douches.

Vaginal dryness has been shown to be reduced by ArginMax for Women. In an adequately designed research study with 77 women, the results showed an increased satisfaction with overall sex life, in addition to a reduction of vaginal dryness.

Estrogen therapy

There are several forms of estrogen therapy:

1. Vaginal estrogen creams such as Estrace, Premarin, and others are inserted directly into the vagina with an applicator, usually at bedtime, two or three times per week. Vaginal estrogen creams should not be used as a lubricant for vaginal intercourse.
2. A plastic estrogen-infused ring, called Estring, is a soft, flexible ring that is inserted into the inner part of the vagina by the woman or her health care practitioner. It resembles a vaginal diaphragm without a center. The ring remains in place for three months, during which time it releases a steady dose of estrogen. It does not interfere with vaginal intercourse.
3. Vagifem is an estrogen tablet that is inserted into the vagina with a disposable applicator. It is usually applied twice per week.

Although the ability of estrogen to stimulate growth of uterine tissue could promote uterine cancer, the amount of estrogen absorbed into the body by the three methods listed above is too low to stimulate significant growth of uterine tissue and is therefore unlikely to be cancer-promoting. Orally administered or higher doses of estrogen, however, can produce undesirable uterine stimulation. To counteract that effect, progesterone, which inhibits uterine growth, is added to the higher-dose estrogen treatments to prevent the growth of uterine tissue.

What causes premature ejaculation?

PREMATURE, RAPID, OR EARLY ejaculation (usually called PE) is one of the most common male sexual disorders. According to some studies, this condition affects one in three men between the ages of eighteen and fifty-nine. Initially, the criterion of PE was the experience of a short latency (one to two minutes) from vaginal penetration to ejaculation. This criterion is now considered inadequate and has been replaced: PE is now defined as a consistent inability to intentionally delay ejaculation.

One of the most common causes of PE involves psychological factors, particularly anxiety. There is commonly an element of distress in both partners. Men who worry about the sexual satisfaction of their partners may have an increased tendency to experience PE.

Although we don't have a full understanding of the neural processes that enable a man to control the timing of his ejaculation and orgasm, the findings from many studies suggest that the neurotransmitter serotonin is involved in this process. This conclusion is based on the frequent observation that men taking SSRI antidepressants (selective serotonin reuptake inhibitors), which increase the level of serotonin in the brain, complain of anorgasmia—indicating that serotonin may delay orgasm. Men taking these same antidepressants for treatment of PE seem to increase the latency—the time it takes to ejaculate—from less than one minute to between two and six minutes.

Although SSRIs have been reported, anecdotally, to be effective in correcting PE, no oral or topical agents, including SSRIs, have been approved by the FDA for the treatment of this problem. One of the criticisms associated with the use of most SSRIs for the treatment of

PE is that they can produce side effects such as dry mouth, nausea, drowsiness, and anorgasmia. It's advisable to consult a psychiatrist or an experienced general practitioner before using any form of antidepressant drugs (including SSRIs) for PE. Some men report that they find one type of SSRI more effective than others. It's important to consult a physician before changing the type or dose of SSRI, or stopping it altogether.

In about one-third of cases, men with PE also show some degree of erectile dysfunction, which typically results in PE without full erection. In these cases, treatment with drugs such as Viagra can be beneficial. Men with PE are often successfully treated with behavioral therapy, including the "stop-start" or "squeeze" techniques, which are based on the idea that PE results from insufficient attention to pre-orgasmic levels of sexual tension.

When PE is associated with a high level of anxiety, moderate amounts of alcohol or a benzodiazepine are reported to be effective in delaying ejaculation. In other cases, the application of a local anesthetic to the glans of the penis (the rounded part at the tip) may significantly prolong ejaculation latency without affecting the quality of orgasm. These local anesthetics, such as lidocaine or prilocaine spray, are typically applied fifteen minutes before intercourse.

Men suffering from PE that is affecting their sex life might be helped by an assessment by a psychosexual therapist, who could then direct them to the most appropriate path for treatment. Sometimes just a course of behavioral psychosexual therapy is sufficient; sometimes medical treatment is necessary. Some of the techniques that are recommended for overcoming PE are: (1) desensitization of the penis, to control the level of excitement elicited by different stimuli from the partner; (2) the squeeze technique, in which the underside of the glans is compressed by the fingers; (3) exercises contracting the muscles of the pelvic floor; and (4) the stop-start technique, in which the penis is stimulated to the point right before ejaculation, then stimulation is stopped for a couple of seconds, then it is repeated. The third time, the man can ejaculate.

Finally, men with PE might simply wear a condom. The condom can prevent oversensitivity of the penis in contact with the vaginal warmth and texture, so the man can enjoy the penetrative sex for a longer time before ejaculating.

How do I have an orgasm while practicing safer sex?

No SEXUAL ACTIVITY—AT LEAST, activity involving two or more people—is completely safe. But there are levels of safety, and you can participate in *safer sex*, taking precautions during sexual activity that can help you avoid acquiring or transmitting an STI. Everyone engaging in sexual activity should understand that STIs are passed around from person to person because the "germs" take advantage of our desire to have sex. The bacteria and viruses that "travel with passion" include genital herpes, HPV (the virus that causes genital warts), HIV, chlamydia, gonorrhea, syphilis, hepatitis B and C, and several others. You can greatly decrease your chances of getting these diseases if you choose to behave in a "safer" manner. It is always important to practice safer sex, and it is extremely important if you and your partner don't know each other's HIV status, have not known each other for a long time, or have been involved in risky health behavior patterns such as having one or more sexual partners, injecting drugs, or sharing needles. Individuals who have had blood transfusions in the past few years, or who are intimate with someone who has, should also be extra cautious. If your partner has been, or may have been, with another partner in the past year, it's wise to use extra protection.

The best way to reduce the possibility of spreading disease when engaging in sexual activity is to avoid the exchange of bodily fluids. Latex condoms, when properly used, greatly reduce (but do not eliminate) the risk of transmitting and receiving an STI. Improper use includes exposing the condom to oils, which break down the latex (oils include Vaseline, massage oil, and many hand creams), and using a condom more than once. However, too many people don't use condoms—and the results of such decisions can be devastating. The reasons people avoid condom use are many. Some men believe that if they use condoms, their partner might think they are having sex with other partners behind her back. Others think that it's unnatural and "impure" to have sex with a barrier. Some couples don't want to interrupt sex to put on the condom. And of course, condoms significantly reduce the pleasurable sensation of direct contact between bare penis and vagina.

Oral sex is much safer when a man wears a condom (unlubricated, to avoid the bad taste). Some couples may prefer dental dams. Dental dams can be used when a woman wants to experience an orgasm from oral sex. The dental dam covers her vulva and clitoris, limiting her exposure to a man's saliva and oral blood. Dental dams and male condoms that are designed for protected oral sex are available in various colors and even different tastes to give more flavor to a couple's sex life.

The first FDA-approved female condom is made of polyurethane, which does not disintegrate with oil-based lubricants. The female condom is usually supplied with lubricant and, like the male condom, should be used only once. Some couples prefer the female condom because it can be inserted hours before sex and so won't interfere with the sexual encounter.

New products are now being developed, called microbicides, which are being tested in animals and humans. These are products that protect against both pregnancy and STIs, including HIV. Women can use these products with a diaphragm or with the Softcup (a feminine hygiene product—*not* itself a contraceptive—known as a menstrual cup), which can be worn for up to 12 hours. Women do not report any change in their orgasmic responses with these products.

Many men participating in studies on condom use and sexual pleasure report that their pleasure decreases when they use condoms, but women don't report the same experience. In fact, some studies show that women whose partners use condoms have more positive attitudes toward sexuality and engage in a higher frequency of sexual activity. This might be because using a well-lubricated condom makes it much easier to penetrate the vagina, which is especially helpful when women experience pain at the beginning of penetration.

Some studies report condom slippage when participants used supplementary lubricant on their condoms for oral and vaginal sexual encounters, so it's advisable to build up the level of supplementary lubricant you use gradually as you become more confident about how to use a condom in this way.

The other benefit of using condoms is that they can help reduce anxiety related to making a mess or impregnation. For a woman, it can help her overcome her fear of contracting an STI or becoming pregnant and may help her relax more, which may help her to experience orgasm. Using a condom may also help her overcome her dislike of pleasuring her partner orally, for fear of ending up with a mouthful of seminal fluid or smelling genital odors.

Can I get HIV/AIDS and other STIs from oral sex?

PROBABLY YES. ORAL SEX, often performed to stimulate an orgasm, is broadly defined as any contact between mouth, lips, and tongue of one person with another person's vulva, penis, or anus. The exact level of risk associated with oral sex is not completely known for each STI because it is very difficult to reliably identify the transmission route of an infection (which may have occurred weeks, months, or years before diagnosis). In one study, 8 of 122 HIV-infected patients (7 percent) were deemed likely to have contracted HIV through oral sex. Researchers in England have also presented conclusive evidence that transmission of HIV can occur from oral sex where the virus travels from penis to mouth, mouth to penis, and vagina to mouth. This risk of acquiring HIV during oral sex is highest for people who have other risk factors such as bleeding disorders, dental problems (loss of a tooth or bleeding gums), and illegal drug use. There is also research showing that the hepatitis B virus can be transferred through oral sex. Some researchers believe that herpes and gonorrhea infections are often transmitted as a result of oral sex. (For safer sex during oral sex, see above, "How do I have an orgasm while practicing safer sex?")

Does diet affect orgasms?

ORGASMS ARE PROBABLY NOT affected very much by our everyday diet. However, since antiquity and in practically all cultures, and still today, there has been a belief that certain foods stimulate sexual desire and performance. In the classical world, men who ate fish, especially salmon, herring, and carp, were thought to have remarkable sexual potency. Other products of the sea, such as ambergris (whale vomit, used as a base for expensive perfumes) and shark fins, were eagerly sought in some cultures as aphrodisiacs. We have found no scientific data in support of the sexual performance–improving effect of the fish diet for men. However, a recent study showed that feeding boars a high diet of omega-3 oil, prevalent in some fish, lengthened the duration of their ejaculation from an already impressive average of 5 minutes 44 seconds to an even more impressive 6 minutes 29 seconds!

Plants, including many herbs, contain a large number of biochemicals that may influence sexual response and orgasm. Since medieval times, garlic, anise, cinnamon, onions, and carrots, among others, have been recommended to cure "anaphrodisia," the lack of sexual interest. However, only a very few of these plant derivatives have been tested in humans and found to have positive effects. One such biochemical is yohimbine, obtained from the tree *Corynanthe yohimbe.* Other herbal products found to have positive effects on sexual response include extracts of *Ginkgo biloba* (maidenhair tree). These extracts contain many potentially active agents known as glycosides, flavonoids, and terpenolactones, which may affect brain regions involved in sexual response. The effect of ginkgo biloba on sexual arousal in men is exerted through relaxation of the smooth muscles of the penis, facilitating erection by increasing blood flow into the penis. Ginkgo biloba has also been reported to counteract the inhibitory effect of antidepressant medication on sexual response, including orgasm, in men and women.

Ginseng is another herbal product that has been reported to improve sexual response. "Ginseng" is a generic term for several plant species belonging to the genus *Panax*. Ginseng contains many biochemicals, including steroids, saponins, and ginsenosides, that may alter the functioning of several of the neurotransmitters—nitric oxide (NO), acetylcholine, and opioids—that are involved in sexual response. Ginseng stimulates penile erection by the pathway that uses nitric oxide as neurotransmitter. The effect on penile erection of these herbal therapies has been confirmed by some studies.

Although no clear information exists on the positive or negative effects of the components of our normal, everyday diet, there is evidence that obesity in men is one cause of erectile dysfunction. Obese men with ED can regain their sexual activity after two years of adopting a "Mediterranean-style" diet, which is rich in fruits, vegetables, nuts, whole grains, and olive oil. The adoption of this type of diet by obese women for a two-year period significantly improved their scores on a rating scale called the "Female Sexual Index." However, whether the diet directly affects a person's sex life or affects weight, which in turn affects sex life, is difficult to evaluate.

Six

The Geography of the Female Orgasm

What is the clitoris?

THE CLITORIS IS A female sex organ located above the vagina. Most people are familiar with the visible head, or glans, of the clitoris. Contact with the glans can heighten a woman's sexual desire and help her experience orgasm. Beneath the glans, the clitoris extends deep into the body and is attached by supporting connective tissues to the pubic bone, mons pubis (a layer of fatty tissue over the pubic bone), labia, urethra, and vagina. The overall shape of the clitoris resembles a thick wishbone, consisting of the visible glans in the midline and two branches, the "bulbs" and the "crura" (singular, "crus").

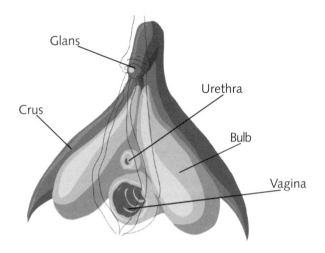

Structure of the clitoris. The clitoris is much larger than just the visible portion (the "glans"). The rest of the clitoris has a wishbone shape that extends deep into the body, straddling the urethra and vagina. Each side of the wishbone consists of a "crus" and a "bulb," both of which are erectile tissues (tissues that can become rigid). These deep components of the clitoris can develop an erection by becoming engorged with blood, similar to what happens in a penis.

What is the cervix?

THE CERVIX, LOCATED AT the far (inner) end of the vagina, is the constricted opening to the uterus. When touched by a finger, it feels somewhat rubbery, like the tip of a nose. Some women say that contact (penis, finger, or sex toy) with the cervix enhances their possibility of experiencing an orgasm and may increase the intensity of their orgasm.

What is the G spot?

THE G SPOT, OR Gräfenberg spot (named by Drs. John Perry and Beverly Whipple for researcher Ernst Gräfenberg, who wrote about this area in 1950), is a sensitive area felt through the front (anterior, belly-side) wall of the vagina about half way between the level of the pubic bone and the cervix (along the course of the urethra). It's easiest to feel the G spot with the woman lying on her back. If one or two fingers are inserted into the vagina, with the palm up, using a "come here" motion, the tissue that surrounds the urethra (through which urine passes from the bladder to the urethral opening) will begin to swell. When the spot is first touched, the woman may feel as if she needs to urinate, but if the touch continues for a few seconds longer, it may turn into a pleasurable feeling. Women have reported that they have difficulty locating and stimulating their G spot by themselves (except with a dildo, a G spot vibrator, or similar device), but they have no difficulty identifying the erotic sensation when the area is stimulated by a partner. To stimulate the G spot during vaginal intercourse, the best positions are the woman on top or rear entry, so the penis will hit the anterior wall of the vagina.

Some women describe experiencing orgasm from stimulation solely of the G spot. The orgasm resulting from stimulation of the G spot is felt deep inside the body, and a bearing-down sensation during the orgasm is commonly reported. Physiologically, the orgasm is different from an orgasm produced by clitoral stimulation. During orgasm with clitoral stimulation, the end of the vagina balloons out. During orgasm from G spot stimulation, the cervix pushes down into the vagina. Many women experience a "blended orgasm" when the G spot and the clitoris are stimulated at the same time. We should note, however, that not all women like the feeling of stimulation of the G spot area.

Some women experience an expulsion of a small amount of fluid (about one teaspoonful) from the urethra with G spot orgasms (as well as with orgasms resulting from stimulation of other areas). The fluid produced by this "female ejaculation" has the appearance of watered-down, fat-free milk. It's chemically similar to seminal fluid and is different from urine. Researcher Milan Zaviacic conducted hundreds of studies on autopsy specimens and concluded that the fluid is from the para-urethral glands, which recently have been named the "female prostate gland." Many men enjoy stimulation of their prostate, which can

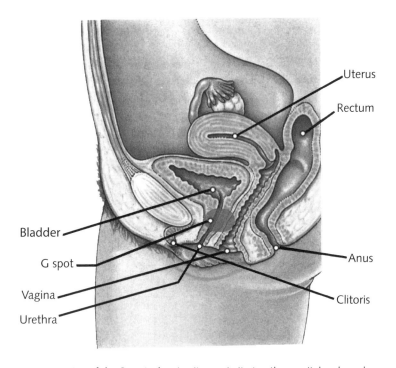

Location of the G spot, showing its proximity to other genital and nearby nongenital structures. (Courtesy Henry Holt and Company)

produce an orgasm that is accompanied by a bearing-down sensation similar to that described by women when they experience an orgasm from G spot stimulation.

Not all researchers have been able to locate the G spot, thus there is some controversy about it. Other researchers consider that the G spot is obvious. It may be that researchers use different methods of stimulation (and thus obtain different results) in studying the G spot area or that not all women have a sensitive G spot area. One group of researchers recently studied twenty women and observed a correlation between vaginal orgasms and the thickness of the "clitoris urethra-vaginal complex also known as the G spot." So, pressure exerted against the anterior vaginal wall may be more effective if the G spot area is thicker, according to this new research. However, the careful terminology (clitoris urethra-vaginal complex) used by the researchers alerts us to the fact that there are several different organs in this highly complex body region. These include (1) the anterior vaginal wall, (2) the urethra, (3) the Skene's glands (also called the para-urethral glands or female prostate gland), (4) perhaps other glands in this region (vestibular glands, Bartholin's glands), (5) the surrounding muscle and connective tissue, and (6) perhaps even portions of the clitoris. The effect of G spot stimulation might primarily be the result of stimulation of just one structure (such as the female prostate gland) or it might be the result of stimulation of several sensitive structures that are close together.

We need to issue a word of caution here. There is a new procedure, called the "G shot," in which a medical doctor injects collagen into the anterior vaginal wall to increase the volume of the G spot region. There are no controlled, scientific studies on this procedure as yet, and nothing about it has been published in peer-reviewed journals. Some women are spending thousands of dollars every four months for something that has not been scientifically documented as effective. We are unable to recommend this expensive procedure.

We suggest that if G spot stimulation feels good, then enjoy it, but don't feel compelled to find it. Some women have been frustrated in their search for their G spot. Regard it as one area of sensual and sexual pleasure that some women enjoy.

What is the U spot?

THE U SPOT HAS been described as a small patch of sensitive erectile tissue located just above and on either side of a woman's urethral opening. It may also include the opening of the urethra. There have been claims that if this region is gently caressed, with the finger, tongue, or tip of the penis, this can produce a particularly strong erotic response. The possible erotic involvement of the U spot was described in Desmond Morris's 2004 book *The Naked Woman: A Study of the Female Body*. To our knowledge, there has not been much study on the role of the U spot in promoting orgasm or erotic sensations.

What is the A spot?

THE A SPOT (MORE technically, the anterior fornix erogenous zone, or AFE zone) was described in the 1990s by Chua Chee Ann, a Malaysian physician, as a possible sexual stimulatory region in women. It's a region of sensitive tissue on the anterior (belly-side) vaginal wall, past the G spot and just before the cervix.

What are the vaginal fornices?

THE ANTERIOR FORNIX, POSTERIOR fornix, and lateral (side) fornix of the vagina are the deepest portions of the vagina. They are the recesses (*fornix* means "arch") created by the slight protrusion of the cervix into the vagina at its inner end. Research has shown that pressure on this area stimulates the vagina to become lubricated. Stimulation of the vaginal fornices can produce orgasmic contractions of the uterus in some women. Women may be able to improve their natural lubrication by stimulating this area.

Seven

Orgasms and Relationships

How can I stimulate or intensify orgasms in myself or my partner?

THERE ARE SEVERAL BASIC strategies you can use to intensify sexual responses and orgasms. Most important to recognize is that our brain is our greatest sexual organ. We can flood it with physical, cognitive, emotional, and pharmacological stimuli that may have additive effects on the intensity of orgasms. For women, combined stimulation of the clitoris, vagina, cervix, nipples, breasts, lips, and personal erogenous zones may intensify the frequency and strength of orgasm. Men describe additive effects on orgasm when penile stimulation is accompanied by stimulation of the scrotum, testicles, prostate, nipples, lips, and personal erogenous zones.

The effects of combined stimulation of these regions are cumulative, because the overall effect on our brain of stimulation of the diverse nerves that carry sensations from these organs may be additive. Combining this physical stimulation with mental imagery and fantasy may intensify the effect still more.

For most people, the ultimate aphrodisiac is true love, with heartfelt and mutual caresses and tenderness. Couples in love almost always report satisfying sexual relationships. Nothing can surpass the delicious fusing of mutual, true love and the passion associated with a nurturing physical relationship. Conversely, nothing leads to a breakdown of both love and the sexual relationship faster than disrespect and betrayal of trust.

How can I tell whether my partner is faking an orgasm?

YOU PROBABLY CAN'T. BOTH men and women do pretend to have orgasms. When doing so, they are probably convinced they will not experience an orgasm and they don't wish their partner to think they are dissatisfied or are incapable of having this pleasurable experience. Faking is dishonest, but we should recognize that the intent is not to harm.

For men, because most of the time an orgasm is followed closely by ejaculation, faking is more difficult. A woman may notice that ejaculation did not occur. For women, orgasm may be experienced on many different levels and may occur with or without external signs. So, it's difficult to tell whether a woman experiences an orgasm or not. Some women have one or more of the following physical indications of orgasm: retraction of the clitoral head (glans), increased breathing and heart rate, dilated pupils, vaginal muscle spasms, skin flushing, and sudden perspiration. However, not everyone shows these responses, and experiencing orgasm is a subjective feeling. The only way to know whether your partner truly has an orgasm is to engage in an honest discussion based on mutual trust.

How can my partner and I have simultaneous orgasms?

Numerous studies have shown that women and men have different experiences leading up to orgasm, especially during penetrative sex. For example, for men, orgasm tends to be experienced as a single peak of intense pleasure, but for women it's often a series of waves of pleasure. Differences in orgasmic pattern, plus individual differences in the time it takes to experience orgasm, create difficulties in attempting to coordinate them.

In Tantric sex, the partners practice gaining control over their excitement, which may help them synchronize and prolong their state of arousal. They learn to read each other's body language and body signals and to be aware of their own and their partner's phase of excitation, which helps them pace their own excitement and pace their erotic stimulation of their partner.

The same principle of paying attention to your partner's state of sexual excitement in relation to your own state is, of course, applicable to all sexual interactions, Tantric or other. By learning your partner's erogenous zones and pattern and timing of excitation, and by heeding your own pattern simultaneously, and with communication, practice, familiarity, and loving tenderness, the likelihood of experiencing orgasms simultaneously is increased. If the woman has prolonged orgasms, one strategy is for the man to wait until she starts to experience an orgasm and then allow himself to experience his orgasm in the midst of hers.

Of course, compulsively setting the goal of "achieving" orgasms simultaneously can be a sure formula for disappointment, frustration, and resentment if that goal is not "attained." Better to heed and learn each other's rhythms and enjoy whatever sexual interaction transpires, whether or not orgasms occur. This strategy may ultimately, unexpectedly, yield the delightful surprise of simultaneous orgasms.

Why does my partner use a vibrator to have an orgasm?

MANY WOMEN SAY THAT they don't experience orgasm through penetrative sex but only through clitoral stimulation. So, although they enjoy vaginal intercourse, they like the simultaneous sensation of clitoral stimulation. This preference may leave a woman's partner in doubt as to whether she enjoys penetrative sex. Good communication—as always—may help dispel the partner's concerns.

Some women enjoy a vibrator's stimulation before or after having penetrative sex with their partner, because women are often physically capable of having several orgasms in succession. Women don't experience the male-typical "refractory period" (a period after orgasm during which an individual can't have another orgasm) and may wish to enjoy the sensation of clitoral stimulation preceding or following penetrative sex. A woman may also prefer the feeling of a vibrator during oral sex, when a man is stimulating her clitoris. The vibrator can be used to stimulate the G spot and other areas.

What can I do if my partner says he can't have an orgasm because my vagina is not tight enough?

THE VAGINA HAS ELASTIC capability—it can dilate to accommodate a baby passing through it and constrict enough to provide friction to a penis. When the male partner says he thinks his partner's vagina is not tight enough, this means that he would prefer greater frictional stimulation of his penis. Surgery of the pelvic region and childbirth may affect the "tightness" of the vagina. Also, some men become used to vigorous penile stimulation when masturbating. In this case, a man could relinquish masturbation and try to sensitize his penis solely to his partner's vagina.

Alternatively, the woman can be more interactive during vaginal intercourse, such as by synchronizing her movements with her partner, and trying to grasp his penis with her pelvic floor muscles. The couple might also experiment with different positions to see which ones provide more intense stimulation.

Kegel exercises to increase the contraction strength of the pelvic floor muscles may provide a tighter grasp of the penis during penetrative intercourse. (For women who wish to try this, we recommend the instructions given at www.mayoclinic.com/health/kegel-exercises/WO 00119. See also "The importance of healthy pelvic muscles," chapter 4 in Ladas, Whipple, and Perry's book *The G Spot and Other Discoveries about Human Sexuality.*)

What can I do if my partner says she isn't having orgasms because my penis is too small?

THE AVERAGE HUMAN PENIS is approximately four to six inches (thirteen to fifteen centimeters) in length when erect. When a woman says her partner's penis is too small, she probably means that she is not getting the stimulation she desires. One of the easiest ways to increase a woman's sensations is to use a textured (such as ribbed) condom.

For some women, increased clitoral stimulation may lead to more satisfying results, while others may prefer the penis to be aimed at their cervix or G spot. The use of a vibrator or dildo may be helpful, if both partners are comfortable with it. These strategies may help reduce the importance of penis size, as alternative forms of pleasurable stimulation are explored.

The woman might try doing Kegel exercises as a way to increase the vaginal grasp of the penis, which will simultaneously increase the intensity of her vaginal stimulation.

The devices and treatments that claim to enlarge a healthy man's penis should be considered with great caution. We are not aware of any research that adequately demonstrates the benefits of such devices or treatments.

Why does my partner want to have an orgasm through anal sex?

"ANAL SEX" TYPICALLY REFERS to insertion of the penis through the anus and into the rectum, but can include anilingus (oral stimulation of the anus), fingering, and use of sex toys, including vibrators and small dildos known as "butt plugs." Some people seek to have anal sex because of the particular pleasure they derive from it. Others may do so for reasons such as avoiding pregnancy or preserving a sense of vaginal virginity.

This form of sexual activity is comparatively high risk, because of the relative ease of tearing the tissue of the anus and rectum, the risk of transmitting viral infections such as HIV, and risks associated with the high bacterial content of the rectum. The tissue lining the rectum provides little natural lubrication, so a personal water-based lubricant is often used with a tear-resistant condom during anal sex.

Some people report experiencing orgasms as a result of anal stimulation. There are probably three different sources of sexual stimulation produced by anal intercourse: sensation from the anus, the rectum, and, in men, the prostate gland. Each of these tissues sends sensory signals to the brain through different pairs of nerves—the anus through the pudendal nerves, the rectum through the pelvic nerves, and the prostate through the hypogastric nerves.

For some men, prostate stimulation produces an orgasm that they describe as "deeper," more global and intense, longer lasting, and associated with greater feelings of ecstasy than orgasm elicited by penile stimulation only. These descriptions of orgasm are similar to women's descriptions of orgasms in response to cervical and uterine stimulation. It's plausible that the similarity in descriptions stems from the fact that the hypogastric nerves transmit sensory stimulation from the cervix and uterus in women and from the prostate gland in men.

In women, orgasms may be elicited from stimulation by way of any of the following nerve routes: from the clitoris through the pudendal nerves, from the vagina and cervix through the pelvic nerves, and from the cervix and uterus through the hypogastric (and probably the vagus) nerves. Stimulation of the G spot region may involve all of these nerves except, perhaps, for the vagus nerves. Because the anus and rectum also send sensory signals to the brain by way of the pudendal and pelvic nerves, respectively, it's likely that these nerves convey the sensory signals that produce orgasm in response to anal and rectal stimulation, both in women and in men.

For those who are interested in engaging in anal sex, it's important to consider your partner's beliefs and comfort level. No one should be pressured or coerced to engage in this type of sex. Because of its relatively high-risk nature, a couple should be committed to a monogamous relationship before considering anal sex. A strong condom that is specifically designed for anal sex should always be used. To avoid injury, perhaps it's advisable to start slowly, massaging the anal region, then inserting fingers to relax the anus, applying generous amounts of lubricant, and advancing gradually.

Why does my partner need me to "talk dirty" in order to have an orgasm?

"Dirty talk" or "talking sexy" is probably arousing because it helps a person fantasize, breaks cultural taboos, or creates a sense of exciting risk-taking. Your partner may find it difficult to experience orgasm without this increased stimulation. Unless there is mutual agreement about this, however, talking sexy runs the risk of offending, insulting, or even turning off one's partner. A higher percentage of men than women find this talk stimulating, although many women do enjoy this type of interaction. Some women seem to get equally or more aroused by hearing endearing and loving words, rather than "dirty talk," during sexual interaction (perhaps related to cultural pressure against their talking about sex). Some research suggests that "dirty talk" might encourage the partners to "act out" their fantasies, leading to unsafe sex practices. Most couples, we hope, have the wisdom to recognize the difference between safe fantasy talk and unsafe real-world experiences.

What can we do if my partner or I can't experience orgasms?

ONE OF THE FIRST things a sexual therapist is taught during training, and will convey to his or her clients, is that orgasm is an *experience*, not a goal. Considered in this context, many people have satisfying sexual experiences without orgasm. While some men and women have tried but have not experienced orgasms, others have never tried and have not felt the need to try. Still others have been orgasmic intermittently, wondering why the experience is not always available to them.

The causes and effects of these situations are likely to be different from one person to another, and they may be cultural, psychological, physiological, or some combination thereof. While there are many similarities between how men and women describe their orgasms, each person may experience orgasms differently and with different forms of stimulation, both physically and mentally. A man may ejaculate without feeling an orgasm or satisfaction, or he may experience orgasm without ejaculating and still derive pleasure and satisfaction from it. Each person is unique and experiences sexual responses in unique ways.

For couples intent on trying to experience orgasm, there are some paths to consider. First, you might start by seeing whether you can stimulate yourself to orgasm. For women, gentle rubbing on the clitoris could be the starting point. If you don't want to touch your genitals, you could use a vibrator or even a flow of water. You could then combine this with stimulating different areas that many women find sensitive, such as the G spot. Try experimenting privately with your own body to see which areas bring you pleasure. This will help you find which combination may feel best and help with your experiencing an orgasm. You could also try stimulating your nipples, which are known to be erogenous for some women. Stimulation of the vaginal entrance also may contribute to erotic feelings.

Once a woman knows what brings her pleasure (even if she has not experienced an orgasm), she can guide her partner (verbally or nonverbally), communicating what she finds stimulating. Of course, the partner must be loving and gentle in such intimate interactions. Remember, nothing is a bigger turnoff than disrespect.

Men who have difficulty experiencing orgasm should probably try self-stimulation first. Stimulation of the penis by hand is usually sufficient. Some men find that stimulation with a vibrator is helpful. Try experimenting with other potential erogenous areas of the body, such as the scrotum, testicles, prostate, and nipples.

Some people feel uncomfortable about self-pleasuring or self-exploration. For these individuals, they might ask their partner to explore their body and discover together how various parts of their body respond to different stimulation. As each partner explores the other's body, comfort, nonverbal communication, and discussion may develop. Make use of the discoveries to give each other pleasure. This may prolong your sex-play time and bring you closer to each other, even if you don't experience orgasm.

Another exercise is to focus on different senses. For example, experiment with different aromas. For women, this could mean wearing a particular perfume that she wears only when in an erotic mood; for men, a particular cologne. Visual stimulation may also increase the chances of experiencing orgasm: a couple might look through an erotic magazine or watch a movie they both find erotic. Couples can play with texture, each partner applying different textures to the other's body to see how they feel, which kind of touch is most relaxing, and which is most arousing. Often it is what couples say or don't say that is the most erotic—try using arousing words or relaxing music. You might want to read to each other from books or poems that you find erotic. Finally, some people find it stimulating to involve food in their romance—feeding each other or putting whipped cream, honey, or chocolate syrup over the body, and then licking it off.

It may be helpful for partners, separately, to write down what they find pleasing, share the results with each other, and then destroy the written record so that the information is seen as very personal. If done with respect, each partner can understand and respond to the desires of the other. If you discover what arouses you and your partner, and use what you learn, it may help you stay focused during sexual experiences and may help you experience an orgasm.

For those who wish to seek help from a professional, the best starting points are the American Association of Sexuality Educators, Counselors and Therapists (AASECT), the Society for Sex Therapy and Research (SSTAR), and the British Association for Sexual and Relationship Therapy (BASRT), all of which have international members. All have a website you can visit.

Eight

Orgasms and Culture

Do different cultures view orgasms differently?

YES, VIEWS OF ORGASM do differ among cultures, which is not surprising. Given the vast diversity of values, attitudes, and practices among the world's many cultures, we would hardly expect sexual behavior to be exempt from cultural interpretations. Yet, historical texts from a variety of cultures eloquently describe pleasurable orgasmic sensations resulting from sexual activity. In most of the world's cultures, discussions concerning how men and women can and should experience sexual pleasure, including orgasm, have been a part of their tradition. Sometimes these discussions are intended to reduce sexual activity (such as the often repeated myths that if a man has orgasms through self-stimulation, he will go blind or grow hair on his palms, or his hand will turn green). At other times, discussions are intended to foster a better marriage—for example, in some Islamic cultures, men are encouraged to withhold ejaculation until they are certain that their wife is satisfied.

We are, each of us, embedded within a culture and influenced by it. Your view of orgasm and the prevailing view in your culture may be aligned or may be in conflict. In this time of growing cross-cultural relationships, we suggest that, for the sake of more fulfilling sexual relationships, each of us should learn as much as possible about our own culture and others (this is particularly important if your partner's culture is different from your own). In this way, each person probably has the best chance of maximizing his or her sexual experiences.

Does female genital cutting affect orgasms?

FEMALE GENITAL CUTTING, OR female genital mutilation (FGM)— also called, inaccurately, female circumcision—is a practice that has been documented among peoples in certain parts of the world, regardless of religion (and including Judaism, Christianity, and Islam). The severity of the procedure depends on differences in locale, educational attainment, and socioeconomic status rather than religious affiliation. Depending on the type of genital cutting and the parts that are injured or removed, women can have a variety of experiences in their sex life, including orgasm. These experiences can range from having no problems to having (1) severe infections, (2) a deep fear of being touched, (3) severe pain during penetrative sex, (4) difficulties during childbirth, and (5) hemorrhaging.

Although some women might undergo genital cutting as an expression of cultural and social conformity, others are coerced or undergo the event as a child. In all cases, the World Health Organization considers female genital cutting a violation of human rights, because it denies women the right to be free from "cruel, inhuman or degrading treatment." The World Health Organization categorizes the types of female genital mutilation as follows:

- Type 1: *Clitoridectomy.* Removal of the prepuce (the hood of the clitoris), with or without all or part of the clitoris.
- Type 2: *Excision.* Removal of the clitoris with partial or total excision of the inner lips (labia minora) of the vulva. The remaining skin may be stitched together.

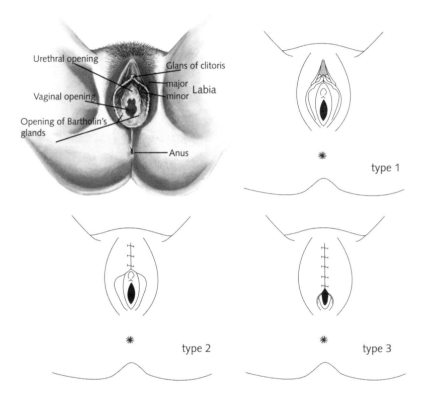

Types of genital cutting. The different types vary in severity. In type 1 (least severe), the hood of the clitoris (prepuce) is removed, with or without all or part of the clitoral glans. In type 2, the glans and part or all of the labia minora are removed, and the remaining skin may be stitched together. In type 3, the glans, labia minora, and labia majora are removed and the remaining skin is stitched together, leaving a small exit hole for urination and menstruation. (Adapted from image courtesy Allison Rogers)

- Type 3: *Infibulation.* Removal of all or part of the clitoris and the inner and outer lips (labia majora) of the vulva. The raw skin is then stitched together, leaving a tiny opening for urination and menstruation. The scar reopens during childbirth and is then re-stitched.
- Type 4: *Other.* Pricking, piercing, cutting, or stretching of the clitoris and/or labia; burning of the clitoris and surrounding tissue; scraping or cutting of the vagina; introduction of corrosive substances or herbs into the vagina to cause bleeding or for the purpose of tightening or narrowing the vagina.

Depending on which body parts have been removed by the genital cutting, women may report pain during intercourse, which may create a fear of intercourse and decrease their sexual activity, frequency of orgasms, and sexual desire. This problem could be partly due to trauma to the nerve supply to the vulva and clitoris. One study compared women who did and women who did not undergo the "less severe" types of genital cutting, and found that 66 percent of the cut women and 59 percent of the uncut women said they usually or always had an orgasm during intercourse. However, the cut women were more likely to cite the breasts than the clitoris as their most sensitive body part. The study's authors concluded that genital cutting does not eliminate a woman's sexual sensation, but instead "shift[s] . . . the point of maximal sexual stimulation from the clitoris . . . or labia to the breasts." Based on the same study, the authors reported that any type of genital cutting can increase the chance of urinary tract infections, itching (pruritus) in the genital area, pain while urinating, and pain during sexual intercourse. So, although this "less severe" type of female genital cutting might not eliminate responsiveness to sexual stimulation, it may be harmful to a woman's reproductive health.

Does male circumcision affect orgasms?

MALE CIRCUMCISION WAS PERFORMED at least as early as 6,000 years ago, as we know from findings in Egyptian mummies. The Bible (Genesis 14) recounts a covenant between God and Abraham, which includes: "and he who is eight days old shall be circumcised among you, every male throughout your generations." This ancient tradition for Jews continues to this day, and it is widely practiced by Christians and Muslims as well. The issue of male circumcision is controversial for some people. There are hygienic arguments for its practice, although researchers disagree on whether or not circumcision reduces the transmission of sexually transmitted infections (STIs).

The ability of a man to experience an orgasm doesn't seem to be greatly affected by circumcision; however, some woman may be affected by male circumcision. Women whose partner has a foreskin may experience increased duration and comfort of sexual intercourse and may have an increased likelihood of experiencing single and multiple orgasms.

Does piercing affect orgasms?

IN A QUESTIONNAIRE STUDY of thirty-three women who responded before and after undergoing voluntary piercing of their clitoral sheath (hood, or prepuce), there was no significant change in their orgasms after piercing. The only significant change was an increase in their "desire." The study had no control group, so it's possible that these women underwent the piercing as a means of fulfilling a wish to increase their desire—which is just a somewhat complicated way of saying that the study was not designed to give foolproof results.

The research team of Miller and Edenholm reported two case studies of female genital piercing. In one, the woman said that the metal ring through her clitoral sheath increased the intensity of clitoral stimulation during intercourse. In the other case, the ring pierced the woman's clitoral sheath and anterior labia minora (a piercing method termed the "triangle"). Before the piercing, she "required masturbation to achieve orgasm. After piercing, orgasm intensity increased, and with intercourse she reached multiple climaxes."

In a survey of many different types of genital piercing in men and women in England, researcher William Anderson and his colleagues provide a colorful lexicon for piercing of the genitals. In men, piercing the pubic skin over the penis—"pubic piercing" or "rhinoceros horn"—is said to enhance the woman's clitoral stimulation during intercourse. In the "ampallang" or "palang," the glans of the penis is pierced horizontally above the urethra. The "apadravya" is the vertical equivalent through the glans, but it pierces the urethra. The "dydoe" pierces the coronal ridge (rim) of the glans. The "frenum" is a single ring piercing of the underside of the glans. In the "frenum ladder," there are multiple (perhaps six) piercings along the underside of the penis. The "Jacob's ladder" is the equivalent, but on the top side of the penis. The "Prince Albert," in which a ring pierces the urethral opening and the undersurface of the penis, is reported to provide "an intense urethral stimulation during intercourse." In the "reverse Prince Albert," the urethral opening and the upper surface of the penis are pierced. The "dragonfly" adds six flexible plastic "wings" to the "Prince Albert," which increases the intensity of vaginal stimulation during intercourse. In the "Prince's wand," a bar is inserted into the urethra and exits through the underside of the penis. The "hafada" is a piercing of the upper part of the scrotum. The "guiche" (rhymes with "quiche") pierces the raphe (seam), the narrow, elevated strip of tissue in the midline that goes from the back of the scrotum to the anus. And last, there is the "anal ring," which pierces the anus.

In women, in addition to the "triangle" described above, there is the large "Christina," which is not very popular. The piercing is through the external portion (glans) of the clitoris rather than the sheath (prepuce) and exits through the abdominal skin above the pubic bone.

Some of the health risks of genital piercing include hepatitis B and C, HIV, bacterial infections, allergic reactions, difficulty with hygiene, scar tissue formation that could obstruct the urethra, trauma to the vagina or anus, a partner choking on swallowed piercings, and tooth damage.

Does "dry sex" affect orgasms?

"Dry sex" refers to a form of sexual practice in a few communities in African countries in which the woman uses an agent to dry out the natural fluids that normally lubricate the vagina. Some studies report that this drying agent is only warm water (for example, in Zaire or Malawi), while others report the use of local herbs for drying. Among the groups who practice dry sex, the timing of the practice and the importance the community attributes to it vary. In Tonga, a village in Zambia, dry sex is mostly practiced by women after giving birth, because they or their male partner prefer a tighter vagina. However, not all women follow this ritual, nor is it widespread in other parts of that local region.

We could not find any scientific studies specifically addressing a positive or negative relation between dry sex and the experience of orgasm by men or women who practice it. It seems likely that a dry vagina will lead to harsher penetration and more painful intercourse, which could interfere with pleasure and orgasm for the woman. The dryness of the vagina could also promote damage to the delicate tissue of the vaginal lining and increase the likelihood of condom breakage, which could put both partners at risk of unwanted pregnancy, STIs, and HIV.

Is there too much emphasis on "achieving" orgasm in some cultures?

If you feel some cultural pressure to "achieve" orgasm, you are certainly not alone. However, as for all pressures, you have complete control over your reaction to sexual pressures. You probably have noticed that in this book we prefer to use the expression "experience orgasm" rather than "achieve orgasm." There is an ongoing debate among medical professionals, sexual psychotherapists, counselors, neuroscientists, physiologists, and other professionals as to whether we should use words such as *achieve, reach, stimulate, elicit, induce,* or *produce* when referring to orgasms.

The disagreement among these professionals is mainly that terms such as *achieving* or *reaching* orgasm can give the impression that sexual activity has orgasm as a goal to be attained, which, if not attained, implies "inadequacy" or even "failure." Neuroscientists and physiologists consider terms such as *elicit, induce, stimulate, generate*, and the like to be neutral, but sexuality professionals tend to view these terms as too coldly "scientific." By contrast, the term *experiencing* orgasm is descriptive yet neutral, avoiding the attitude toward orgasm as a goal to be achieved. A limitation of the word *experiencing* is that it conveys the sense of "being there" while missing the sense of the process, of "getting there," which is at least half of what's important.

Using the term *achieving* orgasm may subtly put pressure on sexual partners to have a goal-oriented sexual relationship, which could lead to disappointment, frustration, and resentment. In movies and TV programs, when a sexual encounter is portrayed, there is typically a point when the partners make the most noise and seem to be at a climax, followed by a relaxation scene. While this may make for entertaining theater, it tends to distort reality, because neither women nor men experience orgasm in every sexual encounter. These cultural exaggerations should be seen as what they are—exaggerations. It's wise not to fall under the influence of unrealistic expectations.

Why can't people talk about orgasms without feeling embarrassed or silly?

MEN AND WOMEN OFTEN have difficulty talking about sex in general, and they may find it even more difficult and embarrassing to talk about orgasm. Fear of seeming naive or improper may cause a defensive reaction—and in that state, many people resort to silliness, joking, sarcasm, or other "detoxifying" strategies that deflect or distract from the issue. Such fear and avoidance of discussing sexual needs, desires, and concerns may compromise an otherwise close relationship. In a long-term relationship, as the couple goes through the life phases of changing health, pregnancy, childbirth, and aging, poor communication about their sexual relationship may create a climate that leads to loss of intimacy, alienation from each other, and deterioration of their relationship.

There is no ideal way for partners to talk with each other about orgasm, but it does seem to help a relationship when the partners communicate their sexual beliefs, feelings, and desires and the intimacy they wish to share when experiencing orgasm. It's obviously not helpful to begin a discussion with a criticism or complaint. Instead, you might begin with a compliment: "I really liked it when you . . ." Or, "You made me feel good when you . . ." Mutual expressions of respect and reassurance can go a long way toward reducing the embarrassment and easing the dialogue with your partner about your orgasms or your desire to experience them. Try to remember that a healthy sexual relationship—with or without orgasms—is to be cherished. As a wise mother once commented to the newlyweds: "Sex occupies just a brief time during your entire lives. But it's an important time."

Selected References

The following references are just a subset of the literature we have relied on over the years and during the writing of this book. We have not attempted to provide a complete list of references, but rather a listing of sources that will serve as a starting point for those readers who wish to delve deeper into the questions raised by our book.

1. About Orgasms

What are orgasms?

Hyde, J. S. 2005. *Biological Basis of Human Sexuality.* Washington, DC: American Psychological Association.

Kinsey, A., Pomeroy, W., Martin, C., & Gebhard, P. 1953. *Sexual Behavior in the Human Female.* Philadelphia: W. B. Saunders.

Komisaruk, B. R., Beyer-Flores, C., & Whipple, B. 2006. *The Science of Orgasm.* Baltimore: Johns Hopkins University Press.

Masters, W., & Johnson, V. 1966. *Human Sexual Response.* Boston: Little, Brown.

Money, J., Wainwright, G., & Hingburger, D. 1991. *The Breathless Orgasm: A Lovemap Biography of Asphyxiophilia.* New York: Prometheus Books.

Do men and women have the same sensations during an orgasm?

Mah, K., & Binik, Y. M. 2005. Are orgasms in the mind or the body? Psychosocial versus physiological correlates of orgasmic pleasure and satisfaction. *Journal of Sex and Marital Therapy* 31:187–200.

Vance, E. B., & Wagner, N. N. 1976. Written descriptions of orgasm: a study of sex differences. *Archives of Sexual Behavior* 5:87–98.

Why don't all my orgasms feel the same?

Alzate, H., & Londoño, M. L. 1984. Vaginal erotic sensitivity. *Journal of Sex and Marital Therapy* 10:49–56.

Cutler, W. B., Zacker, M., McCoy, N., Genovese-Stone, E., & Friedman, E. 2000. Sexual response in women. *Obstetrics and Gynecology* 95(4, suppl. 1):S19.

Jacoby, S. 1999. Great sex: what's age got to do with it? *AARP/Modern Maturity.* www.aarp.org/mmaturity/sept_oct99/greatsex.html.

Komisaruk, B. R., & Whipple, B. 2000. How does vaginal stimulation produce pleasure, pain and analgesia? In *Sex, Gender and Pain*, ed. R. B. Fillingim. Seattle: IASP Press.

Ladas, A. K., Whipple, B., & Perry, J. D. 2005. *The G Spot and Other Discoveries about Human Sexuality.* New York: Owl Books.

What are multiple orgasms?

Chia, M., & Abrams, R. C. 2005. *The Multi-orgasmic Woman.* New York: Rodale Press.

Chia, M., & Arava, D. A. 1996. *The Multi-orgasmic Man.* San Francisco: HarperSanFrancisco.

Hartman, W., & Fithian, M. 1984. *Any Man Can: The Multiple Orgasmic Technique for Every Loving Man.* New York: St. Martin's Press.

Shtarkshall, R. A., Anonymous, & Feldman B. S. 2008. A woman with a high capacity for multi-orgasms: a qualitative non-clinical case report. *Sexual and Relationship Therapy* 23(3):259–270.

Whipple, B., Myers, B., & Komisaruk, B. R. 1998. Male multiple ejaculatory orgasms: a case study. *Journal of Sex Education and Therapy* 23:157–162.

What is anorgasmia?

Basson, R., Leiblum, L., Brotto, L., Derogatis, L., Fourcroy, J., Fugl-Myer, K., Graziottin, A., Heiman, J. R., Laan, E., Meston, C., Schover, L., van Lankfeld, J., & Weijmar Schultz, W. C. M. 2004. Revised definitions of women's sexual dysfunction. *Journal of Sexual Medicine* 1:40–48.

Heiman, J. R. 2007. Orgasmic disorders in women. In *Principles and Practice of Sex Therapy*, 4th ed., ed. S. Leiblum. New York: Guilford Press.

Jones, K. P., Kingsberg, S., & Whipple, B. 2005. *ARHP Clinical Proceedings: Women's Sexual Health in Midlife and Beyond.* Washington, DC: Association of Reproductive Health Professionals.

Lue, T. F., Giuliano, F., Montorsi, F., Rosen, R., Andersson, K. E., Althof, S., Christ, G., Hatzichristou, D., Hirsch, M., Kimoto, Y., Lewis, R., McKenna, K., McMahon, C., Morales, A., Mucahy, J., Padma-Nathan, H., Pryor, J., Saenz de Tejada, I., Shabsigh, R., & Wagner, G. 2004. Summary of the recommendations on sexual dysfunction in men. *Journal of Sexual Medicine* 1:6–23.

Rosen, R. C. 2000. Prevalence and risk factors of sexual dysfunction in men and women. *Current Psychiatry Reports* 2:189–195.

At what age do orgasms begin?

Bancroft, J. 2005. The endocrinology of sexual arousal. *Journal of Endocrinology* 186:411–427.

Ford, C. S., & Beach, F. A. 1951. *Patterns of Sexual Behavior*. New York: Ace Books.

Kinsey, A. C., Pomeroy, W. B., & Martin, C. E. 1948. *Sexual Behavior in the Human Male*. Philadelphia: W. B. Saunders.

Kinsey, A. C., Pomeroy, W. B., Martin, C. E., & Gebhard, P. 1953. *Sexual Behavior in the Human Female*. Philadelphia: W. B. Saunders.

Do orgasms end at a certain age?

Dennerstein, L., Lehert, P., Burger, H., & Dudley, E. 1999. Factors affecting sexual function of women in the mid-life years. *Climacteric* 2:254–262.

Hayes, R., & Dennerstein, L. 2005. The impact of aging on sexual function and sexual dysfunction in women: a review of population-based studies. *Journal of Sexual Medicine* 2:317–330.

Kingsberg, S. A. 2002. The impact of aging on sexual function in women and their partners. *Archives of Sexual Behavior* 31:431–437.

Schill, W. B. 2001. Fertility and sexual life of men after their forties and in older age. *Asian Journal of Andrology* 3:1–7.

Smith, L. J., Mulhall, J. P., Monogahn, N., & Reid, M. C. 2007. Sex after seventy: a pilot study of sexual function in older persons. *Journal of Sexual Medicine* 4:1547–1553.

How long does it take to reach orgasm?

Komisaruk, B. R., Beyer, C., & Whipple, B. 2008. Orgasm. *Psychologist* 21:100–103.

Masters, W., & Johnson, V. 1966. *Human Sexual Response.* Boston: Little, Brown.

Stubbs, K. R. 2004. *Kama Sutra of Sensual Bathing: A Tantric Guide for Lovers.* Tucson, AZ: Secret Garden Publishing.

Waldinger, M. D. 2005. Lifelong premature ejaculation: definition, serotonergic neurotransmission and drug treatment. *World Journal of Urology* 23:102–108.

Waldinger, M. D., & Schweitzer, D. H. 2005. Retarded ejaculation in men: an overview of psychobiological insights. *World Journal of Urology* 23:76–81.

How long do orgasms normally last?

Gil-Vernet, J. M. Jr., Alvarez-Vijande, R., & Gil-Vernet, A. 1994, Ejaculation in men: a dynamic endorectal ultrasonographical study. *British Journal of Urology* 73:442–448.

Masters, W., & Johnson, V. 1966. *Human Sexual Response.* Boston: Little, Brown.

Nagai, A., Watanabe, M., Nasu, Y., Iguchi, H., Kusumi, N., & Kumon, H. 2005. Analysis of human ejaculation using color Doppler ultrasonography: a comparison between antegrade and retrograde ejaculation. *Urology* 65:365–368

How often do people experience orgasm?

Ellis, H. 1910. *Studies in the Psychology of Sex.* London: F. A. Davis.

Ford, C. S., & Beach, F. A. 1951. *Patterns of Sexual Behavior.* New York: Ace Books.

Frank, E., Anderson, C., & Rubenstein, D. 1978. Frequency of sexual dysfunction in normal couples. *New England Journal of Medicine* 299:111–115.

Hawton, K., Gath, D., & Day, A. 1994. Sexual function in a community sample of middle-aged women with partners: effects of age, marital, socioeconomic, psychiatric, gynecological, and menopausal factors. *Archives of Sexual Behavior* 23:375–395.

Kingsberg, S. A. 2002. The impact of aging on sexual function in women and their partners. *Archives of Sexual Behavior* 31:431–437.

Kinsey, A. C., Pomeroy, W. B., & Martin, C. E. 1948. *Sexual Behavior in the Human Male.* Philadelphia: W. B. Saunders.

Does a person inherit the ability to have orgasms?

Dawood, K., Kirk, K. M., Bailey, J. M., Andrews, P. W., & Martin, N. G. 2005. Genetic and environmental influences on the frequency of orgasm in women. *Twin Research and Human Genetics* 8:27–33.

Dunn, K. M., Cherkas, L. F., & Spector, T. D. 2005. Genetic influences on variation in female orgasmic function: a twin study. *Biology Letters* 1:260–263.

Are there really "nongenital" orgasms?

Calleja, J., Carpizo, R., & Berciano, J. 1988. Orgasmic epilepsy. *Epilepsia* 29:635–639.

Komisaruk, B. R., Beyer, C., & Whipple, B. 2006. *The Science of Orgasm.* Baltimore: Johns Hopkins University Press.

Stayton, W. 1980. A theory of sexual orientation: the universe as a turn on. *Topics in Clinical Nursing* 1:1–7.

Stubbs, K. R. 2003. *Erotic Passions.* Tucson, AZ: Secret Garden Publishing.

Whipple, B., Ogden, G., & Komisaruk, B. R. 1992. Physiological correlates of imagery-induced orgasm in women. *Archives of Sexual Behavior* 21:121–133.

Why do people sometimes look as if they are in pain at or near orgasm?

Bodnar, R. J., Commons, K., & Pfaff, D. W. 2002. *Central Neural States Relating Sex and Pain.* Baltimore: Johns Hopkins University Press.

Komisaruk, B. R., Beyer, C., & Whipple, B. 2006. *The Science of Orgasm.* Baltimore: Johns Hopkins University Press.

Komisaruk, B. R., Whipple, B., & Beyer, C. 2009, in press. Sexual pleasure. In *Pleasures of the Brain: Neural Bases of Sensory Pleasure*, ed. K. C. Berridge and M. Kringelbach. New York: Oxford University Press.

2. Women's Orgasms

What's the difference between vaginal, cervical, and clitoral orgasms?

Alzate, H., & Londoño, M. L. 1984. Vaginal erotic sensitivity. *Journal of Sex and Marital Therapy* 10:49–56.

Cutler, W. B., Zacker, M., McCoy, N., Genovese-Stone, E., & Friedman, E. 2000. Sexual response in women. *Obstetrics and Gynecology* 95(4, suppl. 1):S19.

Glenn, J., & Kaplan, E. H. 1968. Types of orgasm in women: a critical review and redefinition. *Journal of the American Psychoanalytic Association* 16:549–564.

Komisaruk, B. R., Beyer, C., & Whipple, B. 2006. *The Science of Orgasm*. Baltimore: Johns Hopkins University Press.

Ladas, A. K., Whipple, B., & Perry, J. D. 1982. *The G Spot and Other Recent Discoveries about Human Sexuality*. New York: Holt, Rinehart and Winston.

Does breast or nipple stimulation affect a woman's orgasm?

Kayner, C. E., & Sager, J. A. 1983. Breast feeding and sexual response. *Journal of Family Practice* 17:69–73.

Kinsey, A., Pomeroy, W., Martin, C., & Gebhard, P. 1953. *Sexual Behavior in the Human Female*. Philadelphia: W. B. Saunders.

Masters, W., & Johnson, V. 1966. *Human Sexual Response*. Boston: Little, Brown.

Paget, L. 2001. *The Big O*. New York: Broadway Books.

Do Kegel exercises intensify female orgasms?

Barbach, L. G. 1975. *For Yourself: The Fulfillment of Female Sexuality*. New York: Doubleday.

Graber, B. 1982. *Circumvaginal Musculature and Sexual Function*. New York: Karger.

Graber, B., & Kline-Graber, G. 1979. Female orgasm: role of the pubococcygeus. *Journal of Clinical Psychiatry* 40:348–351.

Kegel, A. H. 1952. Sexual functions of the pubococcygeus muscle. *Western Journal of Surgery, Obstetrics, and Gynecology* 60:521–524.

Perry, J. D., & Whipple, B. 1981. Pelvic muscle strength of female ejaculators: evidence in support of a new theory of orgasm. *Journal of Sex Research* 171:22–39.

What fluids are produced before and during a woman's orgasm?

Belzer, E. G., Whipple, B., & Moger, W. 1984. On female ejaculation. *Journal of Sex Research* 20:403–406.

Cabello, F. 1997. Female ejaculation: myths and reality. In *Sexuality and Human Rights*, ed. J. J. Borras-Valls & M. Perez-Conchillo. Valencia, Spain: Nau Libres.

Gräfenberg, E. 1950. The role of the urethra in female orgasm. *International Journal of Sexology* 3:145–148.

Ladas, A. K., Whipple, B., & Perry, J. D. 1982. *The G Spot and Other Recent Discoveries about Human Sexuality.* New York: Holt, Rinehart and Winston.

Whipple, B., & Komisaruk, B. R. 1991 The G spot, vaginal orgasm and female ejaculation: a review of research and literature. In *Proceedings of the First International Conference on Orgasm*, ed. P. Kothari and R. Patel. Bombay: VRP Publishers.

Zaviacic, M. 1999. *The Human Female Prostate: From Vestigial Skene's Paraurethral Glands and Ducts to Woman's Functional Prostate.* Bratislava, Slovakia: Slovak Academic Press.

Why is the clitoris so sensitive after an orgasm?

Gruenwald, I., Lowenstein, L., Gartman, I., & Vardi, Y. 2007. Physiological changes in female genital sensation during sexual stimulation. *Journal of Sexual Medicine* 4:390–394.

Levin, R., & Riley, A. 2007. The physiology of human sexual function. *Psychiatry* 6:90–94.

Vardi, Y., Gruenwald, I., Sprecher, E., Gertman, I., & Yartnitsky, D. 2000. Normative values for female genital sensation. *Urology* 56:1035–1040.

Does body position during sex affect a woman's orgasm?

Eichel, E. W., Eichel, J. D., & Kule, S. 1988. The technique of coital alignment and its relation to female orgasmic response and simultaneous orgasm. *Journal of Sex and Marital Therapy* 14:129–141.

Ladas, A. K., Whipple, B., & Perry, J. D. 1982/2005. *The G Spot and Other Discoveries about Human Sexuality*. New York: Holt.

Whipple, B., & Welner, S. L. 2004. Sexuality issues. In *Welner's Guide to the Care of Women with Disabilities*, ed. S. L. Welner & F. Hazeltine. Philadelphia: Lippincott, Williams & Wilkins.

Does penis size affect a woman's orgasm?

Eisenman, R. 2001. Penis size: survey of female perceptions of sexual satisfaction. *BMC Women's Health* 1:1.

Francken, A. B., van de Wiel, H. B. M., van Driel, M. F., & Weijmar Schultz, W. C. M. 2002. What importance do women attribute to the size of the penis? *European Urology* 42:426–431.

Mondaini, N., Ponchietti, R., Gontero, P., Muir, G. H., Natali, A., Caldarera, E., Biscioni, S., & Rizzo, M. 2002. Penile length is normal in most men seeking penile lengthening procedures. *International Journal of Impotence Research* 14:283–286.

Tiefer, L., Pedersen, B., & Melman, A. 1988. Psychosocial follow-up of penile prosthesis implant patients and partners. *Journal of Sex and Marital Therapy* 14:184–201.

Are orgasms affected by the menstrual cycle?

Cutler, W. B., Friedmann, E., & McCoy, N. L. 1996. Coitus and menstruation in perimenopausal women. *Journal of Psychosomatic Obstetrics and Gynecology* 17:149–157.

Filer, R. B., & Wu, C. H. 1989. Coitus during menses: its effect on endometriosis and pelvic inflammatory disease. *Journal of Reproductive Medicine* 34:887–890.

Heiman, J. R., & LoPiccolo, J. 1999. *Becoming Orgasmic: A Sexual and Personal Growth Programme for Women*. London: Piatkus.

Meaddough, E. L., Olive, D. L., Gallup, P., Perlin, M., & Kliman, H. J. 2002. Sexual activity, orgasm and tampon use are associated with a decreased risk for endometriosis. *Gynecologic and Obstetric Investigation* 53:163–169.

Morris, N. M., & Udry, J. R. 1983. Menstruation and marital sex. *Journal of Biosocial Science* 15:173–181.

Is a woman more likely to become pregnant if she has an orgasm?

Baker, R. R., & Bellis, M. A. 1995. *Human Sperm Competition: Copulation, Masturbation and Infidelity.* London: Chapman and Hall.

Fox, C. A., Wolff, H. S., & Baker, J. A. 1970. Measurement of intra-vaginal and intra-uterine pressures during human coitus by radio-telemetry. *Journal of Reproduction and Fertility* 22:243–251.

Lloyd, E. A. 2005. *The Case of the Female Orgasm: Bias in the Science of Evolution.* Cambridge, MA: Harvard University Press.

Wildt, L., Kissler, S., Licht, P., & Becker, W. 1998. Sperm transport in the human female genital tract and its modulation by oxytocin as assessed by hysterosalpingoscintigraphy, hysterotonography, electrohysterography and Doppler sonography. *Human Reproduction Update* 4:655–666

Is it safe to have orgasms during pregnancy?

Chhabra, S., & Verma, P. 1991. Sexual activity and onset of preterm labour. *Indian Journal of Maternal and Child Health* 2:54–55.

Ekwo, E. E., Gosselink, C. A., Woolson, R., Moawad, A., & Long, C. R. 1993. Coitus late in pregnancy: risk of preterm rupture of amniotic sac membranes. *American Journal of Obstetrics and Gynecology* 168:22–31.

Petridou, E., Salvanos, H., Skalkidou, A., Dessypris, N., Moustaki, M., & Trichopoulos, D. 2001. Are there common triggers of preterm deliveries? *BJOG: An International Journal of Obstetrics and Gynaecology* 108:598–604.

Sayle, A. E., Savitz, D. A., Thorp, J. M. Jr., Hertz-Picciotto, I., & Wilcox, A. J. 2001. Sexual activity during late pregnancy and risk of preterm delivery. *Obstetrics and Gynecology* 97:283–289.

von Sydow, K. 1999. Sexuality during pregnancy and after childbirth: a meta-content-analysis of 59 studies. *Journal of Psychosomatic Research* 47:27–49.

Does childbirth affect orgasm?

Barrett, G., Pendry, E., Peacock, J., Victor, C., Thakar, R., & Manyonda, I. 2000. Women's sexual health after childbirth. *BJOG: An International Journal of Obstetrics and Gynaecology* 107:186–195.

Hall, K. 2004. *Reclaiming Your Sexual Self: How You Can Bring Desire Back into Your Life.* New York: Wiley.

Harel, D. 2007. Sexual experiences of women during childbirth. Unpublished doctoral dissertation. San Francisco: The Institute for Advanced Study of Human Sexuality.

Martyn, E. 2001. *Baby Shock! Your Relationship Survival Guide.* London: Relate.

Signorello, L. B., Bernard, L., Harlow, A., Chekos, K., & Repke, J. T. 2001. Postpartum sexual functioning and its relationship to perineal trauma: a retrospective cohort study of primiparous women. *American Journal of Obstetrics and Gynecology* 184:881–890.

von Sydow, K. 1999. Sexuality during pregnancy and after childbirth: a meta-content-analysis of 59 studies. *Journal of Psychosomatic Research* 47:27–49.

How do hormones affect women's orgasms?

Abdallah, R. T., & Simon, J. A. 2007. Testosterone therapy in women: its role in the management of hypoactive sexual desire disorder. *International Journal of Impotence Research* 19:458–463.

Bancroft, J. 2005. The endocrinology of sexual arousal. *Journal of Endocrinology* 186:411–427.

Kingsberg, S. 2007. Testosterone treatment for hypoactive sexual desire disorder in postmenopausal women. *Journal of Sexual Medicine* 4(suppl. 3):227–234.

Schmidt, P. J., Steinberg, E. M., Negro, P. P., Haq, N., Gibson, C., & Rubinow, D. R. 2009. Pharmacologically induced hypogonadism and sexual function in healthy young women and men. *Neuropsychopharmacology* 34:565–576.

Traish, A., Guay, A. T., Spark, R. F., & Testosterone Therapy in Women Study Group. 2007. Are the Endocrine Society's clinical practice guidelines on androgen therapy in women misguided? A commentary. *Journal of Sexual Medicine* 4:1223–1235.

3. Men's Orgasms

How does a penis become erect?

Argiolas, A., & Melis, M. R. 2005. Central control of penile erection: role of the paraventricular nucleus of the hypothalamus. *Progress in Neurobiology* 76:1–21.

Lue, T. F. 2000. Erectile dysfunction. *New England Journal of Medicine.* 342:1802–1813.

Steers, W. D. 2000. Neural pathways and central sites involved in penile erection: neuroanatomy and clinical implications. *Neuroscience and Biobehavioral Reviews* 24:507–516.

How do men ejaculate?

Coolen, L. M., Allard, J., Truitt, W. A., & McKenna, K. E. 2004. Central regulation of ejaculation. *Physiology and Behavior* 83:203–215.

Levin, R. J. 2005. The mechanisms of human ejaculation: a critical analysis. *Sexual and Relationship Therapy* 20:123–131.

McKenna, K. E. 2005. The central control and pharmacological modulation of sexual function. In *Biological Substrates of Human Sexuality*, ed. J. S. Hyde. Washington, DC: American Psychological Association.

Shafik, A. 2000. Mechanism of ejection during ejaculation: identification of a urethrocavernosus reflex. *Archives of Andrology* 44:77–83.

Steers, W. D. 2000. Neural pathways and central sites involved in penile erection: neuroanatomy and clinical implications. *Neuroscience and Biobehavioral Reviews* 24:507–516.

Does a penis need to be hard to have an orgasm?

Brindley, G. S. 1983. Physiology of erection and management of paraplegic infertility. In *Male Infertility*, ed. T. B. Hargreave. New York: Springer-Verlag.

Why is the penis so sensitive after an orgasm?

Kim, D. S., Lee, J. Y., & Pang, M. G. 2002. Male circumcision: a South Korean perspective. *BJU International* 83(S1):28–33.

Levin, R., & Riley, A. 2007. The physiology of human sexual function. *Psychiatry* 6:90–94.

Rowland, D. L., Haensel, S. M., Blom, J. H. M., & Slob, K. 1993. Penile sensitivity in men with premature ejaculation and erectile dysfunction. *Journal of Sex and Marital Therapy* 19:189–197.

Waldinger, M. D., Quinn, P., Dilleen, M., Mundayat, R., Schweitzer, D. H., & Boolell, M. 2005. A multinational population survey of intravaginal ejaculation latency time. *Journal of Sexual Medicine* 2:492–497.

Can a man have an orgasm without stimulation of his penis?

Kinsey, A., Pomeroy, W., & Martin, C. 1948. *Sexual Behavior in the Human Male.* Philadelphia: W. B. Saunders.

Can men experience ejaculation without orgasm, or orgasm without ejaculation?

Csoka, A., Bahrick, A., & Mehtonen, O. P. 2008. Persistent sexual dysfunction after discontinuation of selective serotonin reuptake inhibitors. *Journal of Sexual Medicine* 5:227–233.

Ishak, W. W., Berman, D. S., & Peters, A. 2008. Male anorgasmia treated with oxytocin. *Journal of Sexual Medicine* 5:1022–1024.

Kuriansky, J. 2002. *The Complete Idiot's Guide to Tantric Sex.* Indianapolis: Alpha Books.

Levin, R. 2003. Is prolactin the biological "off switch" for human sexual aousal? *Sexual and Relationship Therapy* 18:237–243.

Tamam, Y., Tamam, L., Akil, E., Yasan, A., & Tamam, B. 2008. Post-stroke sexual functioning in first stroke patients. *European Journal of Neurology* 15:660–666.

Why do some men become so sleepy after an orgasm?

Argiolas, A., & Melis, M. R. 2003. The neurophysiology of the sexual cycle. *Journal of Endocrinological Investigation* 26(suppl.):20–22.

Masters, W. H., & Johnson, V. E. 1963. The sexual response of the human male: I. Gross anatomic considerations. *Western Journal of Surgery, Obstetrics, and Gynecology* 71:85–95.

Xue-Rui, T., Ying, L., Da-Zhong, Y., & Xiao-Jun, C. 2008. Changes of blood pressure and heart rate during sexual activity in healthy adults. *Blood Pressure Monitoring* 13:211–217.

What is the clear fluid that comes out of the penis before ejaculation?

Chughtal, B., Sawas, A., O'Malley, R., Nahik, R. R., Ali Kan, S., & Pentyala, S. 2005. A neglected gland: a review of Cowper's gland. *International Journal of Andrology* 28:745–777.

Zukerman, Z., Weics, D. B., & Orvieto, R. 2003. Does preejaculatory penile secretion originating from Cowper's gland contain sperm? *Journal of Assisted Reproduction and Genetics* 20:157–159.

What is the difference between semen and sperm?

Mann, T., & Lutwak-Mann, C. 1981. *Male Reproductive Function and Semen*. New York: Springer-Verlag.

Prins, G. S. 1999. Semen. In *Encyclopedia of Reproduction*, vol. 4. New York: Academic Press.

Zaneveld, L. J. D., & Chatterton, R. T. 1982. *Biochemistry of Mammalian Reproduction*. New York: Wiley

Why does semen change from opaque to transparent?

de Lamirande, E. 2007. Semenogelin, the main protein of the human semen coagulum, regulates sperm function. *Seminars in Thrombosis and Hemostasis* 33:60–68.

Waheed, A., Hassan, M. I., Etten, R. L., & Ahmad, F. 2008. Human seminal proteinase and prostate-specific antigen are the same protein. *Journal of Biosciences* 33:195–207.

Wang, Z. J., Zhang, W., Feng, N. H., Song, N. H., Wu, H. F., & Sui, Y. G. 2008. Molecular mechanism of epididymal protease inhibitor modulating the liquefaction of human semen. *Asian Journal of Andrology* 10:770–775

What causes differences in the amount and characteristics of semen ejaculated?

Filippi, S., Vignozzi, L., Vannelli, G. B., Ledda, F., Forti, G., & Maggi, M. 2003. Role of oxytocin in the ejaculatory process. *Journal of Endocrinological Investigation* 26:82–86.

Holstege, G. 2005. Central nervous system control of ejaculation. *World Journal of Urology* 23:109–114.

Kollberg, S., Petersen, I., & Stener, I. 1962. Preliminary results of an electromyographic study of ejaculation. *Acta Chirurgica Scandinavica* 123:478–483.

Shafik, A. 1997. Pelvic floor muscles and sphincters during erection and ejaculation. *Archives of Andrology* 39:71–78.

Shafik, A., & El-Sibai, O. 2000. Mechanism of ejection during ejaculation: identification of a urethrocavernosus reflex. *Archives of Andrology* 44:77–83.

How do hormones affect men's orgasms?

Beyer, C., Morali, G., Larsson, K., & Sodersten, P. 1976. Steroid regulation of sexual behavior. *Journal of Steroid Biochemistry* 7:1171–1176.

Komisaruk, B. R., Beyer, C., & Whipple, B. 2006. *The Science of Orgasm*. Baltimore: Johns Hopkins University Press.

O'Connor, D. B., Archer, J., & Wu, F. C. 2004. Effects of testosterone on mood, aggression, and sexual behavior in young men: a double-blind, placebo-controlled, cross-over study. *Journal of Clinical Endocrinology and Metabolism* 89:2837–2845.

Reyes-Vallejo, L., Lazarou, S., & Morgentaler, A. 2007. Subjective sexual response to testosterone replacement therapy based on initial serum levels of total testosterone. *Journal of Sexual Medicine* 4:1757–1762.

Steidle, G., Schwartz, S., Jocoli, K., Sebree, T., Smith, T., & Bachand, R. 2003. AA2500 testosterone gel normalizes androgen levels in aging males with improvements in body composition and sexual function. *Journal of Clinical Endocrinology and Metabolism* 88:2673–2681.

4. Hows and Whys of Orgasm

How do legal and illegal drugs affect orgasm?

Baldwin, D. S. 2004. Sexual dysfunction associated with antidepressant drugs. *Expert Opinion on Drug Safety* 3:457–470.

Basson, R. 2001. Female sexual response: the role of drugs in the management of sexual dysfunction. *Obstetrics and Gynecology* 98:350–353.

Clayton, D. O., & Shen, W. W. 1998. Psychotropic drug-induced sexual function disorders: diagnosis, incidence and management. *Drug Safety* 19:299–312.

Shen, W. W., & Soto, L. S. 1990. Inhibited female orgasm resulting from psychotropic drugs: a five year updated clinical review. *Journal of Reproductive Medicine* 35:11–14.

Why do people sometimes experience orgasms while asleep?

Brissette, S., Montplaisir, J., Godbout, R., & Lavoisier, P. 1985. Sexual activity and sleep in humans. *Biological Psychiatry* 20:758–763.

Fisher, C., Cohen, H. D., Schiavi, R. C., Davis, D., Furman, B., Ward, K., Edwards, A., & Cunningham, J. 1983. Patterns of female sexual arousal during sleep and waking: vaginal thermo-conductance studies. *Archives of Sexual Behavior* 12:97–122.

Money, J. 1960. Phantom orgasm in the dreams of paraplegic men and women. *Archives of General Psychiatry* 3:373–382.

Why do people say that orgasms happen in the brain?

Georgiadis, J. R., Kortekaas, R., Kuipers, R., Nieuwenburg, A., Pruim, J., Reinders, A. A., & Holstege, G. 2006. Regional cerebral blood flow changes associated with clitorally induced orgasm in healthy women. *European Journal of Neuroscience* 24:3305–3316.

Komisaruk, B. R., & Whipple, B. 2005. Functional MRI of the brain during orgasm in women. *Annual Review of Sex Research* 16:62–86.

Komisaruk, B. R., Whipple, B., & Beyer, C. 2008. Orgasm. *Psychologist* (UK) 21:100–103.

Komisaruk, B., Whipple, B., Crawford, A., Grimes, S., Liu, W.-C., Kalnin, A., & Mosier, K. 2004. Brain activation during vaginocervical self-stimulation and orgasm in women with complete spinal cord injury. *Brain Research* 1024:77–88.

How does "sex-change" ("transsexual") surgery affect orgasms?

Christopher, A. N., & Ralph, D. J. 2008. Total phallic reconstruction. In *Textbook of Reconstructive Urologic Surgery*, ed. D. Montague, I. Gill, K. Angermeier, & J. H. Ross. New York: Taylor & Francis.

Jarolim, L. 2000. Surgical conversion of genitalia in transsexual patients. *BJU International* 85:851–856.

Kim, S. K., Park, J. H., Lee, K. C., Park, J. M., Kim, J. T., & Kim, M. C. 2003. Long-term results in patients after rectosigmoid vaginoplasty. *Plastic and Reconstructive Surgery* 112:143–151.

Krege, S., Bex, A., Lummen, G., & Rubben, H. 2001. Male-to-female transsexualism: a technique, results and long-term follow-up in 66 patients. *BJU International* 88:396–402.

How do machines and devices stimulate orgasms?

Billups, K., Berman, J., Berman, L., Metz, M., Glennon, M., & Goldstein, I. 2001. A new non-pharmacological vacuum therapy for female sexual dysfunction. *Journal of Sex and Marital Therapy* 27:435–441.

Blank, J. 1994. Toys: sex toys. In *Human Sexuality: An Encyclopedia*, ed. V. L. Bullough & B. Bullough. New York: Garland.

Wilson, S., Delk, J., & Billups, K. 2001. Treating symptoms of female sexual arousal disorder with the "Eros-Clitoral Therapy Device." *Journal of Gender Specific Medicine* 4:54–58.

How can scientists tell whether animals have orgasms?

Dixson, A. F. 1998. *Primate Sexuality: Comparative Studies of the Prosimians, Monkeys, Apes and Human Beings*. New York: Oxford University Press.

Fox, C. A., & Fox, B. 1971. A comparative study of coital physiology, with special reference to the sexual climax. *Journal of Reproduction and Fertility* 24:319–336.

Marson, G. A., Nappi, R. P., Pfaus, J., Traish, A. M., Vardi, Y., & Goldstein, I. 2004. Physiology of female sexual function: animal models. *Journal of Sexual Medicine* 1:237–253.

5. Orgasms and Health

Are orgasms good for our health?

Abramov, L. A. 1976. Sexual life and sexual frigidity among women developing acute myocardial infarction. *Psychosomatic Medicine* 386:418–425.

Charnetski, C. J., & Brennan, F. X. 2001. *Feeling Good Is Good for You: How Pleasure Can Boost Your Immune System and Lengthen Your Life*. Emmaus, PA: Rodale Press.

Komisaruk, B. R., Beyer-Flores, C., & Whipple, B. 2006. *The Science of Orgasm*. Baltimore: Johns Hopkins University Press.

Leitzmann, M. F., Platz, E. A., Stampfer, M. J., Willett, W. C., & Giovannucci, E. 2004. Ejaculation frequency and subsequent risk of prostate cancer. *Journal of the American Medical Association* 291:1578–1586.

Whipple, B., Koch, P. B., Moglia, R. F., & Samuels, H. 2007. The health benefits of sexual expression. www.plannedparenthood.org/resources/research-papers/sexual-expression-6358.htm.

Do orgasms reduce stress?

Brody, S., & Krüger, T. H. 2006. The post-orgasmic prolactin increase following intercourse is greater than following masturbation and suggests greater satiety. *Biological Psychology* 713:312–315.

Charnetski, C. J., & Brennan, F. X. 2001. *Feeling Good Is Good for You: How Pleasure Can Boost Your Immune System and Lengthen Your Life.* Emmaus, PA: Rodale Press.

Komisaruk, B. R., & Whipple, B. 1998. Love as sensory stimulation: physiological effects of its deprivation and expression. *Psychoneuroendocrinology* 23:927–944.

Planned Parenthood Federation of America. 2007. *The Health Benefits of Sexual Expression.* White paper published in cooperation with the Society for the Scientific Study of Sexuality. New York: Katharine Dexter McCormick Library.

Sanderson, C. 2006. *Counselling Adult Survivors of Child Sexual Abuse.* London: Jessica Kingsley Publishers.

Can an orgasm cause a heart attack?

Fairchild, K. A., & Whipple, B. 2001. Addressing sexual concerns of women with heart disease. *Medical Aspects of Human Sexuality* 1:35–39.

Feldman, H. A., Johannes, C. B., McKinlay J. B., & Longcope, C. 1998. Low dehydroepiandrosterone sulfate and heart disease in middle-aged men: cross-sectional results from the Massachusetts Male Aging Study. *Annals of Epidemiology* 8:217–228.

Garner, W. E., & Allen, H. A. 1989. Sexual rehabilitation and heart disease. *Journal of Rehabilitation* 55:69–73

Green, A. W. 1975. Sexual activity and the postmyocardial infarction patient. *American Heart Journal* 89:246–252.

Safi, A. M., & Stein, R. A. 2001. Cardiovascular risks of sexual activity. *Current Psychiatry Reports* 3:209–214.

Can orgasms cause headaches?

Evans, R. W., & Couch, J. R. 2001. Orgasm and migraine. *Headache* 41:512–514.

Frese, A., Gantenbein, A., Marziniak, M., Husstedt, I. W., Goadsby, P. J., & Evers, S. 2006. Triptans in orgasmic headache. *Cephalalgia: An International Journal of Headache* 26:1458–1461.

Paulson, G. W., & Klawans, H. L. 1974. Benign orgasmic cephalgia. *Headache* 13:181–187.

Valenca, M. M., Valenca, L. P. A. A., Bordini, C. A., Farias da Silva, W., Leite, J. P., Antunes-Rodrigues, J., & Speciali, J. G. 2004. Cerebral vasospasm and headache during sexual intercourse and masturbatory orgasms. *Headache* 44:244–248.

What causes "blue balls"?

Chalett, J. M., & Nerenberg, L. T. 2000. "Blue balls": a diagnostic consideration in testiculoscrotal pain in young adults. A case report and discussion. *Pediatrics* 106:843.

Chalett, J. M., & Nerenberg, L. T. 2001. In reply. *Pediatrics* 108:1234–1235.

Ludovici, L. N., & Arndt, J. 2005. The true cause of blue balls. http://pediatrics.aappublications.org/cgi/eletters/108/5/1233.

Rockney, R., & Alario, A. J. 2001. Blue balls. *Pediatrics* 108:1233–1234.

Weinzimer, S. A., & Thornton, P. S. 2001. To the editor. *Pediatrics* 108:1234.

What is the effect of cancer and its treatment on orgasm?

Beckjord, E., & Campas, B. E. 2007. Sexual quality of life in women with newly diagnosed breast cancer. *Journal of Psychosocial Oncology* 25:19–36.

Chorost, M. I., Weber, T. K., Lee, R. J., Rodriguez-Biqas, M. A., & Petrelli, N. J. 2000. Sexual dysfunction, informed consent and multimodality therapy for rectal cancer. *American Journal of Surgery* 179:271–274.

Ganz, P. A., Greendale, G. A., Petersen, L., Zibecchi, L., Kahn, B., & Belin, T. R. 2000. Managing menopausal symptoms in breast cancer survivors: results of a randomized controlled trial. *Journal of the National Cancer Institute* 92:1054–1064.

Schover, L. R. 1997. *Sexuality and Fertility after Cancer.* New York: John Wiley & Sons.

Does hysterectomy affect orgasms?

Farrell, S. A., & Kieser, K. 2000. Sexuality after hysterectomy. *Obstetrics and Gynecology* 95:1045–1050.

Goetsch, M. F. 2005. The effect of total hysterectomy on specific sexual sensations. *American Journal of Obstetrics and Gynecology* 192:1922–1927.

Maas, C. P., Weijenborg, P. T., & ter Kuile, M. M. 2003. The effect of hysterectomy on sexual functioning. *Annual Review of Sex Research* 14:83–113.

Mokate, T., Wright, C., & Mander, T. 2006. Hysterectomy and sexual function. *Journal of the British Menopause Society* 12:153–157.

Besides hysterectomy, do other female genital surgeries affect orgasms?

Jensen, P. T., Groenvold, M., Klee, M. C., Thranov, I., Petersen, M. A., & Machin, D. 2004. Early-stage cervical carcinoma, radical hysterectomy, and sexual function. *Cancer* 100:97–106.

Rogers, R. G., Kammerer-Doak, D., Darrow, A., Murray, K., Olsen, A., Barber, M., & Qualls, C. 2004. Sexual function after surgery for stress urinary incontinence and/or pelvic organ prolapse: a multicenter prospective study. *American Journal of Obstetrics and Gynecology* 191:206–210.

Schmidt, C. E., Bestmann, B., Kuchler, T., Longo, W. E., & Kremer, B. 2005. Ten-year historic cohort of quality of life and sexuality in patients with rectal cancer. *Diseases of the Colon and Rectum* 48:483–492.

Does prostate surgery affect orgasms?

Koeman, M., van Driel, M. F., Weijmar Schultz, W. C. M., & Mensink, H. J. A. 1996. Orgasm after radical prostatectomy. *British Journal of Urology* 77:861–864.

Miranda-Sousa, A. J., Davila, H. H., Lockhart, J. L., Ordorica, R. C., & Carrion, R. E. 2006. Sexual function after surgery for prostate or bladder cancer. *Cancer Control* 13:179–187.

Nehra, A., Grantmyre, J., Nadel, A., Thibonnier, M., & Brock, G. 2005. Vardenafil improved patient satisfaction with erectile hardness, orgasmic function and sexual experience in men with erectile dysfunction following nerve sparing radical prostatectomy. *Journal of Urology* 173:2067–2071.

Schover, L. R. 2005. Sexuality and fertility after cancer. *Hematology: American Society of Hematology Education Program*, 523–527.

Besides prostate surgery, do other male genital surgeries affect orgasms?

Feldman, H. A., Goldstein, I., Hatzichristou, D. G., Krane, R. J., & McKinlay, J. B. 1994. Impotence and its medical and psychological correlates: results of the Massachusetts Male Aging Study. *Journal of Urology* 151:54–61.

Gandhi, N., Purandare, N., & Lock, M. 1993. Surgical castration for sex offenders: boundaries between surgery and mutilation are blurred. *British Medical Bulletin* 307:1141.

Hendren, S., O'Connor, B., Liu, M., Asano, T., Cohen, Z., Swallow, C., MacRae, H., Gryfe, R., & McLeod, R. 2005. Prevalence of male and female sexual dysfunction is high following surgery for rectal cancer. *Annals of Surgery* 242:212–223.

Are there surgeries that can improve a man's chance of experiencing orgasm?

Lue, T. F. 2000. Erectile dysfunction. *New England Journal of Medicine* 342:1802–1813.

Ringert, R. H., Hermanns, M., & Zoeller, G. 1999. Outcome after repair of congenital penile malformations. *Andrologia* 31(suppl. 1):21–26.

Smith, J. F., Walsh, T. J., & Turek, P. J. 2008. Ejaculatory duct obstruction. *Urology Clinics of North America* 35:221–227.

How do brain injuries or spinal cord injuries affect orgasms?

Chapelle, P. A., Durand, J., & Lacert, P. 1980. Penile erection following complete spinal cord injury in man. *British Journal of Urology* 52:216–219.

Komisaruk, B. R., Gerdes, C. A., & Whipple, B. 1997. "Complete" spinal cord injury does not block perceptual responses to genital self-stimulation in women. *Archives of Neurology* 54:1513–1520.

Komisaruk, B., & Whipple, B. 2006. Neurological impairment of sexuality in men and women. In *Sexual Health*, ed. M. Tepper and A. Owens, vol. 2. Westport, CT: Praeger.

Sipski, M. L., Alexander, C. J., & Rosen, R. 2001. Sexual arousal and orgasm in women: effects of spinal cord injury. *Annals of Neurology* 49:35–44.

Whipple, B., & Komisaruk, B. R. 1997. Sexuality and women with complete spinal cord injury. *Spinal Cord* 35:136–138.

What treatments are there for erectile dysfunction?

Claes, H., & Baert, L. 1993. Pelvic floor exercise versus surgery in the treatment of impotence. *British Journal of Urology* 711:52–57.

Ito, T., Kawahara, K., Das, A., & Strudwick, W. 1998. The effects of ArginMax, a natural dietary supplement for enhancement of male sexual function. *Hawaii Medical Journal* 57:741–744.

Lue, T. F. 2000. Erectile dysfunction. *New England Journal of Medicine* 342:1802–1813.

Lue, T. F., Giuliano, F., Montorsi, F., Rosen, R., Andersson, K. E., Althof, S., Christ, G., Hatzichristou, D., Hirsch, M., Kimoto, Y., Lewis, R., McKenna, K., McMahon, C., Morales, A., Mucahy, J., Padma-Nathan, H., Pryor, J., Saenz de Tejada, I., Shabsigh, R., & Wagner, G. 2004. Summary of the recommendations on sexual dysfunction in men. *Journal of Sexual Medicine* 1:6–23.

Rosen, R. C. 2000. Medical and psychological interventions for erectile dysfunction: toward a combined treatment approach. In *Principles and Practice of Sex Therapy*, ed. S. R. Leiblum and R. C. Rosen. New York: Guilford Press.

Does Viagra help women experience orgasm?

Caruso, S., Intelisano, G., Farina, M., Di Mari, L., & Agnello, C. 2003. The function of sildenafil on female sexual pathways: a double blind, cross-over, placebo-controlled study. *European Journal of Obstetrics, Gynecology, and Reproductive Biology* 110:201–206.

Komisaruk, B. R., Beyer-Flores, C., & Whipple, B. 2006. *The Science of Orgasm.* Baltimore: Johns Hopkins University Press.

Sipski, M. L., Rosen, R. C., Alexander, C. J., & Hamer, R. M. 2000. Sildenafil effects on sexual and cardiovascular responses in women with spinal cord injury. *Urology* 55:812–815.

Does vaginal dryness affect orgasms?

Bachmann, G. A. 1995. Influence of menopause on sexuality. *International Journal of Fertility and Menopausal Studies* 40(suppl.):16–22.

Ito, T. Y., Polan, M. L., Whipple, B., & Trant, A. S. 2006. The enhancement of female sexual function with ArginMax, a nutritional supplement, among women differing in menopausal status. *Journal of Sex and Marital Therapy* 32:369–378.

Van der Laak, J. A. W. M., de Bie, L. M. T., de Leeuw, H., de Wilde, P. C. M., & Hansellar, A. G. J. M. 2002. The effect of Replens® on vaginal cytology in the treatment of postmenopausal atrophy: cytomorphology versus computerized cytometry. *Journal of Clinical Pathology* 556:446–451.

What causes premature ejaculation?

Rowland, D. L., Haensel, S. M., Blom, J. H. M., & Slob, K. 1993. Penile sensitivity in men with premature ejaculation and erectile dysfunction. *Journal of Sex and Marital Therapy* 19:189–197.

Waldinger, M. D. 2005. Lifelong premature ejaculation: definition, serotonergic neurotransmission and drug treatment. *World Journal of Urology* 23:102–108.

Wang, W. F., Wang, Y., Minhas, S., & Ralph, D. J. 2007. Can sildenafil treat primary premature ejaculation? A prospective clinical study. *International Journal of Urology* 14:331–335.

How do I have an orgasm while practicing safer sex?

Khan, S. I, Hudson-Rodd, N., Saggers, S., Bhuiyan, M. I., & Bhuiya, A. 2004. Safer sex or pleasurable sex? Rethinking condom use in the AIDS era. *Sexual Health* 14:217–225.

Randolph, M. E., Pinkerton, S. D., Bogart, L. M., Cecil, H., & Abramson, P. R. 2007. Sexual pleasure and condom use. *Archives of Sexual Behavior* 36:844–848.

Sanders, S. A., Graham, C. A., Yarber, W. L., Crosby, R. A., Dodge, B., & Milhausen, R. R. 2006. Women who put condoms on male partners: correlates of condom application. *American Journal of Health Behavior* 305:460–466.

Whipple, B., & Ogden, G. 1989. *Safe Encounters: How Women Can Say Yes to Pleasure and No to Unsafe Sex.* New York: McGraw-Hill/Pocket Books.

Can I get HIV/AIDS and other STIs from oral sex?

Dillon, B., Hecht, F. M., Swanson, M., Goupil-Sormany, I., Grant, R. M., Chesney, M. A., & Kahn, J. O. 2000. Primary HIV infections associated with oral transmission. Paper presented at Seventh Conference on Retroviruses and Opportunistic Infections, San Francisco, January 30–February 2. Abstract 473.

Gerbert, B., Herzig, K., Volberding, P., & Stansell, J. 1999. Perceptions of health care professionals and patients about the risk of HIV transmission through oral sex: a qualitative study. *Patient Education and Counseling* 381:49–60.

Keet, I. P., Albrecht van Lent, N., Sandfort, T. G., Coutinho, R. A., & van Griensven, G. J. 1992. Orogenital sex and the transmission of HIV among homosexual men. *AIDS* 62:223–226.

Public Health Agency of Canada. 2004. Oral sex and the risk of HIV transmission. HIV/AIDS Epi Update. May. www. phac-aspc.gc.ca/publicat.

Robinson, E. K., & Evans, B. G. 1999. Oral sex and HIV transmission. *AIDS* 13:737–738.

Does diet affect orgasms?

Cohen, A. J., & Bartlik, B. 1998. Ginkgo biloba for antidepressant-induced sexual dysfunction. *Journal of Sex and Marital Therapy* 24:139–143.

Ito, T., Kawahara, K., Das, A., & Strudwick, W. 1998. The effects of ArginMax, a natural dietary supplement for enhancement of male sexual function. *Hawaii Medical Journal* 57:741–744.

Rowland, D. L., & Tai, W. 2003. A review of plant derived and herbal approaches to the treatment of sexual dysfunction. *Journal of Sex and Marital Therapy* 29:185–205.

Spinella, M. 2001. *The Psychopharmacology of Herbal Medicines*. Cambridge, MA: MIT Press.

6. The Geography of the Female Orgasm

What is the clitoris?

O'Connell, H. E., Eizenberg, N., Rahman, M., & Cleeve, J. 2008. The anatomy of the distal vagina: towards unity. *Journal of Sexual Medicine* 5:1883–1891.

O'Connell, H. E., Sanjeevan, K. V., & Hutson, J. M. 2005. Anatomy of the clitoris. *Journal of Urology* 174:1189–1195.

What is the cervix?

Komisaruk, B. R., Beyer-Flores, C., & Whipple, B. 2006. *The Science of Orgasm.* Baltimore: Johns Hopkins University Press.

Komisaruk, B., Whipple, B., Crawford, A., Grimes, S., Liu, W.-C., Kalnin, A., & Mosier, K. 2004. Brain activation during vaginocervical self-stimulation and orgasm in women with complete spinal cord injury. *Brain Research* 1024:77–88.

What is the G spot?

Gravina, G. L., Brandetti, F., Martini, P., Caros, E., DiStasi, S. M., Morano, S., Lenzi, A., & Jannini, E. A. 2008. Measurement of the thickness of the urethrovaginal space in women with or without vaginal orgasm. *Journal of Sexual Medicine* 5:610–618.

Ladas, A. K., Whipple, B., & Perry, J. D. 1982/2005. *The G Spot and Other Discoveries about Human Sexuality*. New York: Holt.

Whipple, B. 2000. Ernst Gräfenberg: from Berlin to New York. *Scandinavian Journal of Sexology* 32:43–49.

Whipple, B., & Komisaruk, B. R. 1991 The G spot, vaginal orgasm and female ejaculation: a review of research and literature. In *Proceedings of the First International Conference on Orgasm*, ed. P. Kothari and R. Patel. Bombay: VRP Publishers.

Zaviacic, M. 1999. *The Human Female Prostate: From Vestigial Skene's Paraurethral Gland and Ducts to Woman's Functional Prostate*. Bratislava, Slovakia: Slovak Academic Press.

What is the U spot?

Morris, D. 2004. *The Naked Woman: A Study of the Female Body*. London: Jonathan Cape.

What is the A spot?

Chua Chee, A. 1993. The AFE Zone-G Spot Stimulation Technique: a new method for the treatment of female sexual dysfunction. In *Proceedings of the XI World Congress of Sexology*, ed. I. Charam & G. Lopes. Rio de Janeiro, Brazil.

Chua Chee, A. 1997. A proposal for a radical new sex therapy technique for the management of vasocongestive and orgasmic dysfunction in women: the AFE Zone Stimulation Technique. *British Journal of Sexual and Marital Therapy* 124:357–370.

What are the vaginal fornices?

Alzate, H., & Londoño, M. L. 1984. Vaginal erotic sensitivity. *Journal of Sex and Marital Therapy* 10:49–56.

Kobayashi, A., & Behringer, R. R. 2003. Developmental genetics of the female reproductive tract in mammals. *Nature Reviews Genetics* 4:969–980.

7. Orgasms and Relationships

How can I stimulate or intensify orgasms in myself or my partner?

Dodson, B. 2002. *Orgasms for Two: The Joy of Partner Sex*. New York: Harmony Books.

Ladas, A. K., Whipple, B., & Perry, J. D. 1982/2005. *The G Spot and Other Discoveries about Human Sexuality*. New York: Holt.

Margolis, J. 2004. *O: The Intimate History of the Orgasm*. New York: Grove/ AtlanticSmart Sex Films. www.SexSmartFilms.com.

How can I tell whether my partner is faking an orgasm?

Basson, R. 2003. Biopsychosocial models of women's sexual response: applications to management of desire disorders. *Sex and Relationship Therapy* 18:107–115.

Masters, W., & Johnson, V. 1966. *Human Sexual Response*. Boston: Little, Brown.

Sand, M., & Fisher, W. A. 2007. Women's endorsement of models of female sexual response: the nurses' sexuality study. *Journal of Sexual Medicine* 4:708–719.

How can my partner and I have simultaneous orgasms?

Basson, R. 2000. The female sexual response: a different model. *Journal of Sex and Marital Therapy* 26:51–65.

Dodson, B. 2002. *Orgasms for Two: The Joy of Partnersex*. New York: Harmony Books.

Kuriansky, J. 2001. *The Complete Idiot's Guide to Tantric Sex*. Indianapolis: Alpha Books, Penguin Group U.S.A.

Ladas, A. K., Whipple, B., & Perry, J. D. 1982/2005. *The G Spot and Other Discoveries about Human Sexuality*. New York: Holt.

Why does my partner use a vibrator to have an orgasm?

Cutler, W. B., Zacker, M., McCoy, N., Genovese-Stone, E., & Friedman, E. 2000. Sexual response in women. *Obstetrics and Gynecology* 95(4, suppl. I):S19.

What can I do if my partner says he can't have an orgasm because my vagina is not tight enough?

Braun, V., & Kitzinger, C. 2001. The perfectible vagina: size matters. *Culture, Health and Sexuality* 3:263–277.

Ladas, A. K., Whipple, B., & Perry, J. D. 1982/2005. *The G Spot and Other Discoveries about Human Sexuality*. New York: Holt.

Meston, C. M., Hull, E., Levin, R. J., & Sipski, M. 2004. Disorders of orgasm in women. *Journal of Sexual Medicine* 11:66–68.

Pardo, J. S., Solà, V. D., Ricci, P. A., Guiloff, E. F., & Freundlich, O. K. 2006. Colpoperineoplasty in women with a sensation of a wide vagina. *Acta Obstetrica Gynecologica Scandinavica* 859:1125–1127.

What can I do if my partner says she isn't having orgasms because my penis is too small?

Son, H., Lee, H., Huh, J. S., Kim, S. W., & Paick, J. S. 2003. Studies on self-esteem of penile size in young Korean military men. *Asian Journal of Andrology* 5:185–189.

Stulhofer, A. 2006. How unimportant is penis size for women with heterosexual experience? *Archives of Sexual Behavior* 35:5–6.

Wessells, H., Lue, T. F., & McAninch, J. W. 1996. Penile length in the flaccid and erect states: guidelines for penile augmentation. *Journal of Urology* 156:995–997.

Wylie, K. R., & Eardley, I. 2007. Penile size and the "small penis syndrome." *BJU International* 99:1449–1455.

Why does my partner want to have an orgasm through anal sex?

Anal sex. 2006. http://en.wikipedia.org/wiki/Anal_sex (accessed August 30, 2008).

Baldwin, J. I., & Baldwin, J. D. 2000. Heterosexual anal intercourse: an understudied, high-risk sexual behavior. *Archives of Sexual Behavior* 294:357–373.

Mah, K., & Binik, Y. M. 2001. The nature of human orgasm: a critical review of major trends. *Clinical Psychology Review* 21:823–856.

Morin, J. 1998. *Anal Pleasure and Health: A Guide for Men and Women*. San Francisco: Down There Press.

Why does my partner need me to "talk dirty" in order to have an orgasm?

Adelman, M. B. 1992. Sustaining passion: eroticism and safe-sex talk. *Archives of Sexual Behavior* 21:481–494.

What can we do if my partner or I can't experience orgasms?

American Association of Sexuality Educators, Counselors and Therapists. www .aasect.org.

Dodson, B. 1987. *Sex for One: The Joy of Self-Loving.* New York: Crown Books.

Heiman, J. R., & LoPiccolo, J. 1999. *Becoming Orgasmic: A Sexual and Personal Growth Programme for Women.* London: Piatkus.

Schoen, M. *A Heterosexual Couple Guide to Sexual Pleasure.* A self-help DVD. Produced and directed by Mark Schoen. www.sexsmartfilms.com.

Zilbergeld, B. 1999. *The New Male Sexuality.* New York: Bantam Books.

8. Orgasms and Culture

Do different cultures view orgasms differently?

Ali, K. 2006. *Sexual Ethics and Islam: Feminist Reflections on Qur'an, Hadith and Jurisprudence.* Oxford: Oneworld Publications.

Alpert, R. 2003. Sex in Jewish law and culture. In *Sexuality and the World's Religions,* ed. D. W. Machacek & M. M. Wilcox. Santa Barbara, CA: ABC-CLIO.

Flaherty, A., Gaviria, F. M., Pathak, D., Mitchell, T., Wintrob, R., Richman, J., & Birz, S. 1988. Developing instruments for cross-cultural psychiatric research. *Journal of Nervous and Mental Disease* 176:257–263.

Hidayatullah, A. 2003. Islamic conceptions of sexuality. In *Sexuality and the World's Religions,* ed. D. W. Machacek & M. M. Wilcox. Santa Barbara, CA: ABC-CLIO.

Janssen, D. F. 2007. First stirrings: cultural notes on orgasm, ejaculation, and wet dreams. *Journal of Sex Research* 44:122–134.

Levin, R. J. 2008. Female orgasm: correlation of objective physical recordings with subjective experience. *Archives of Sexual Behavior* 37:855.

Lidke, J. S. 2003. A union of fire and water: sexuality and spirituality in Hinduism. In *Sexuality and the World's Religions,* ed. D. W. Machacek & M. M. Wilcox. Santa Barbara, CA: ABC-CLIO.

Does female genital cutting affect orgasms?

Ali, K. 2006. *Sexual Ethics and Islam,* chap. 6. Oxford: Oneworld Publications.

Baasher, T. 1979. Psychological aspects of female circumcision. In *Traditional Practices Affecting the Health of Women and Children*. WHO/EMRO Technical Publication No. 2. Alexandria, Egypt: World Health Organization.

Baron, E. M., & Denmark, F. L. 2006. An explanation of female genital mutilation. *Annals of the New York Academy of Sciences* 1087:339–355.

Catania, L., Abdulcadir, O., Puppo, V., Verde, J. B., Abdulcadir, J., & Abdulcadir, D. 2007. Pleasure and orgasm in women with female genital mutilation/cutting (FGM/C). *Journal of Sexual Medicine* 4:1666–1678.

el-Defrawi, M. H., Lotfy, G., Dandash, K. F., Refaat, A. H., & Eyada, M. 2001. Female genital mutilation and its psychosexual impact. *Journal of Sex and Marital Therapy* 27:465–473.

World Health Organization. 2008. *Female Genital Mutilation*. Fact Sheet No. 241. www.who.int/mediacentre/factsheets/fs241/en.

Does male circumcision affect orgasms?

Bleustein, C. B., Fogarty, J. D., Eckholdt, H., Arezzo, J. C., & Melman, A. 2005. Effect of neonatal circumcision on penile neurologic sensation. *Urology* 65:773–777.

O'Hara, K., & O'Hara, J. 1999. The effect of male circumcision on the sexual enjoyment of the female partner. *BJU International* 83(suppl. 1):79–84.

Sorrells, M. L., Snyder, J. L., Reiss, M. D., Eden, C., Milos, M. F., Wilcox, N., & Van Howe, R. S. 2007. Fine-touch pressure thresholds in the adult penis. *BJU International* 99:864–869.

Woodward, L. T. 1963. *The History of Surgery*, p. 8. Derby, CT: Monarch.

Does piercing affect orgasms?

Anderson, W. R., Summerton, D. J., Sharma, D. M., & Holmes, S. A. 2003. The urologist's guide to genital piercing. *BJU International* 91:245–251.

Miller, L., & Edenholm, M. 1999. Genital piercing to enhance sexual satisfaction. *Obstetrics and Gynecology* 93:837.

Millner, V. S., Eichold, B. H. II, Sharpe, T. H., & Sherwood, C. L. Jr. 2005. First glimpse of the functional benefits of clitoral hood piercings. *American Journal of Obstetrics and Gynecology* 193:675–676.

Does "dry sex" affect orgasms?

Brown, J. E., Ayowa, O. B., & Brown, R. C. 1993. Dry and tight: sexual practices and potential AIDS risk in Zaire. *Social Science and Medicine* 378:989–994.

Civic, D., & Wilson, D. 1996. Dry sex in Zimbabwe and implications for condom use. *Social Science and Medicine* 42:91–98.

McNamara, R. 1997. Female genital health and the risk of HIV transmission. In *AIDS in Africa and the Caribbean*, ed. G. C. Bond, J. Kreniske, I. Susser, & J. Vincent. Boulder, CO: Westview Press.

Is there too much emphasis on "achieving" orgasm in some cultures?

Barbach, L. 1982. *For Each Other: Sharing Sexual Intimacy*. New York: Anchor Press/ Doubleday.

Barbach, L. 2001. *For Yourself: The Fulfillment of Female Sexuality*. New York: Signet Books.

Why can't people talk about orgasms without feeling embarrassed or silly?

Litvinoff, S. 1999. *The Relate Guide to Sex in Loving Relationships*. Vermilion, England: Realte.

Haavio-Mannila, E., & Kontula, O. 1997. Correlates of increased sexual satisfaction. *Archives of Sexual Behavior* 26:399–419.

Purnine, D. M., & Carey, M. P. 1997. Interpersonal communication and sexual adjustment: the role of understanding and agreement. *Journal of Consulting and Clinical Psychology* 65:1017–1025.

About the Authors

Barry R. Komisaruk, Ph.D., is a Distinguished Service Professor in the Department of Psychology, Rutgers University, and an adjunct professor in the Department of Radiology, the University of Medicine and Dentistry of New Jersey. Supported by federal, state, and foundation grant funding, he has published more than 145 research papers and three books.

Beverly Whipple, Ph.D., R.N., FAAN, is a certified sexuality educator, sexuality counselor, and sexuality researcher, and Professor Emerita at Rutgers University. She has published more than 160 research papers and coauthored six books, one of which, *The G Spot*, has been translated into nineteen languages and was an international bestseller. For its fiftieth anniversary, *The New Scientist* named her one of the fifty most influential scientists in the world.

Sara Nasserzadeh, Ph.D., MSC, Mphil, DIP PST, is a couples counselor, licensed psychosexual therapist, and sexuality researcher. She is a member of the standardization committee of the World Association for Sexual Health, and she lectures widely. Her call-in radio program, *Whispers*, won the BBC World Service Award for the Innovation of the Year 2007.

Carlos Beyer-Flores, Ph.D., is head of the Laboratorio CIRA-Universidad Autónoma de Tlaxcala and a professor of CINVESTAV, Mexico. He has published more than two hundred research papers and was awarded the coveted National Prize in Natural Science of the Mexican government.